RESVER

unleashing the benefits of red wine

Beth Geisler

Healthy Living Publications
Summertown Tennessee

Library of Congress Cataloging-in-Publication Data

Geisler, Beth.
    Resveratrol / Beth Geisler.
        p. ; cm.
    Includes bibliographical references and index.
    ISBN 978-1-57067-242-2
    1. Resveratrol. I. Title.
    [DNLM: 1. Plant Extracts--therapeutic use. 2. Stilbenes. QV 766]
    RM666.R45G45 2011
    615'.321—dc22

                                        2010045842

Book Publishing Company is a member of Green Press Initiative. We chose to print this title on paper with 100% post consumer recycled content, processed without chlorine, which save the following natural resources:

26 trees

716 pounds of solid waste

11,788 gallons of water

2,448 pounds of greenhouse gases

8 million BTU of energy

For more information on Green Press Initiative, visit www.greenpressinitiative.org.

Environmental impact estimates were made using the Environmental Defense Fund Paper Calculator. For more information visit www.papercalculator.org.

Printed on recycled paper

Printed in Canada

Published by Healthy Living Pulbications,
an imprint of Book Publishing Company
P.O. Box 99
Summertown, TN 38483
888-260-8458
www.bookpubco.com

ISBN 13: 978-1-57067-242-2

17 16 15 14 13 12 11   9 8 7 6 5 4 3 2 1

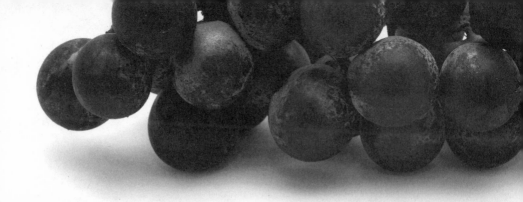

Contents

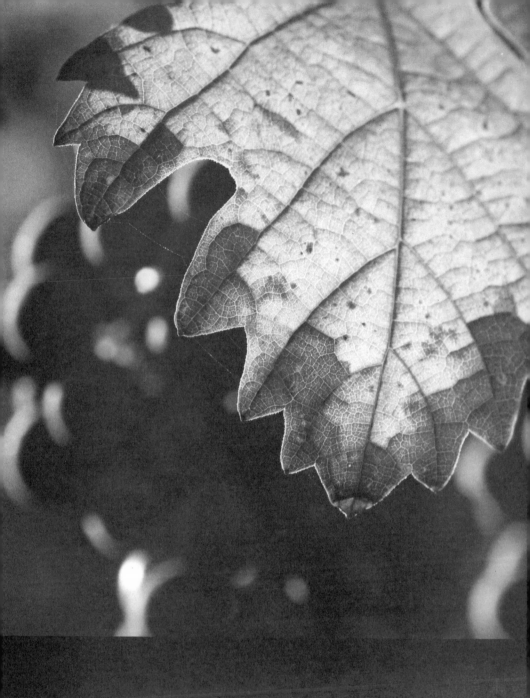

Salute per centánni.

Italian toast wishing good health
for one hundred years

Introduction

ave you heard it through the grapevine? The word is out about the possible health benefits of resveratrol, a chemical found in red wine and certain foods and now available in supplement form. Many studies have shown that resveratrol can prevent or delay the onset of cancer, cardiovascular disease, neurological and brain disorders, diabetes, and viral infection.

Resveratrol may also have the potential to help us live longer, making it a prominent subject in aging and longevity research. In fact, resveratrol has been shown to mimic the healthful effects of calorie restriction, the only proven method for extending life.

In the early 1990s, epidemiologists were surprised when they observed that the French, who eat a high-fat diet, had the lowest incidence of heart disease in Europe. This phenomenon is known as the "French paradox." Because French people traditionally drink wine with meals, one plausible explanation for the French paradox is the high level of resveratrol in red wine. The discovery of the French paradox led to extensive scientific studies designed to discover which specific compounds of red wine had the greatest health-promoting properties.

The health benefits of red wine have been established through a large body of scientific research. One or two glasses a day are considered fine for most adults. People who don't drink red wine can find resveratrol in other sources, such as grape juice, resveratrol-rich foods, and resveratrol supplements. Many of the studies described in this book used laboratory animals who were given megadoses of resveratrol, far more than we could ever get from sipping a glass of red wine, however pleasant that might be.

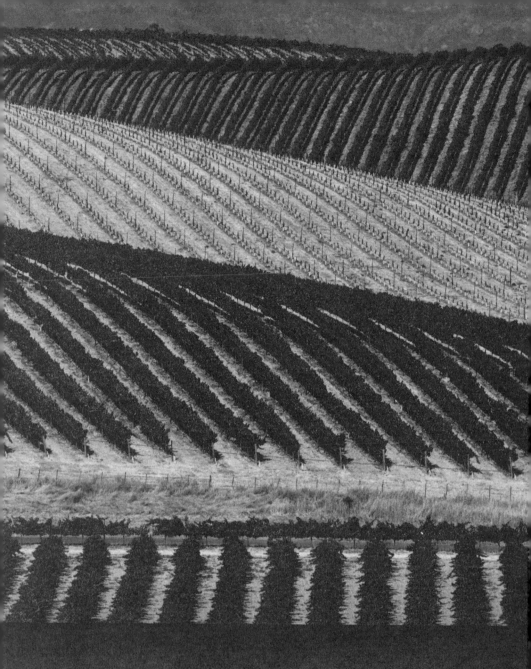

Our food should be our medicine.
Our medicine should be our food.

Hippocrates, physician in ancient Greece

Resveratrol and Antioxidants

R esveratrol is found in more than seventy plant species, primarily in red grapes and red wine, peanuts, some berries, dark chocolate and other cocoa products, and Japanese knotweed (*Polygonum cuspidatum*). Resveratrol was discovered by a Japanese researcher in 1940 and was first isolated from the roots of Japanese knotweed, commonly used in traditional Chinese and Japanese herbal medicine, in 1963. Today, scientific research shows that resveratrol appears to boost heart health, inhibit the growth of cancer cells, and slow aging, in addition to playing a positive role in preventing a host of chronic and degenerative diseases. Recent research has even demonstrated that resveratrol can increase blood flow to the brain.

The most widely recognized source of resveratrol is red wine. In grapes, resveratrol is found mainly in the skins. Red wine contains more resveratrol because the grapes are fermented with the skins longer than for white wine. In fact, resveratrol amounts in these two different types of wine vary substantially. In 2009, Amsterdam researchers published results of a study that measured the resveratrol content in various wines. They found that red wine contains ten to twenty times more resveratrol than white wine, and rosé wine contains only slightly higher concentrations than white.

Resveratrol is a phytoalexin, meaning it is part of a plant's defense arsenal. Grapevines and other plants that produce resveratrol do so because they are stressed when fighting enemies, such as cold or other weather extremes, drought, fungal attack, and injury. These

Japanese Knotweed: Not Just a Weed

Although the name may not be familiar, you have very likely seen Japanese knotweed, which, true to its name, grows like a weed in many parts of North America. In fact, Japanese knotweed is classified as an invasive plant. Although gardeners combat this ubiquitous plant, it is edible and provides important nutrients. Its taste is sometimes compared to rhubarb. Tender spring shoots can be steamed like asparagus, sautéed in oil with garlic, or juiced in a juicer with fruit. Most important, Japanese knotweed is the primary source of resveratrol for dietary supplements.

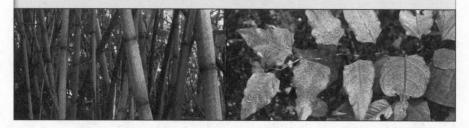

plants generate resveratrol to aid their very chances of survival. Now we are learning that this natural substance that protects plants can protect us as well.

Free Radicals

I f resveratrol is the hero of our story, free radicals are unavoidable villains. Free radicals are atoms or molecules with unpaired electrons that contribute to diseases, including cancer. Substances found

TABLE 1. Resveratrol content in foods

Food	Serving size	Total resveratrol
Red grapes	1 cup (160 g)	0.24–1.25 mg
Peanuts, boiled	1 cup (180 g)	0.32–1.28 mg
Peanut butter	1 cup (258 g)	0.04–0.13 mg
Peanuts, raw	1 cup (146 g)	0.01–0.26 mg

Source: Linus Pauling Institute, Oregon State University. Micronutrient Information Center. http://lpi.oregonstate.edu/infocenter/phytochemicals/resveratrol.

in our environment—like herbicides, pollution, and radiation—cause extraordinary amounts of free radicals in our bodies.

Other free radicals also occur normally. For example, sometimes our immune systems purposefully create them to neutralize viruses and bacteria. Although we have little control over many sources of free radicals, we can limit our exposure to some extent.

Over time, free radicals accumulate in cells. In medicine, the presence and effect of free radicals on our health is called oxidative stress, which is associated with high levels of LDL (low-density lipoprotein), or "bad," cholesterol and artery damage that leads to heart attack and stroke. By damaging our cells and tissues until they can no longer function properly, free radicals threaten our health and hasten our aging. To understand how they accomplish this, let's review some basic high-school chemistry.

In science, the term "radical" refers to a group of atoms or molecules that act together. They contain a nucleus, protons, and electrons. Electrons orbit the nucleus and are involved in chemical reactions. A substance that has a full outer shell of electrons is said to be stable and not interested in combining. However, if the outer ring of electrons is incomplete, the atom will combine with a molecule and take the electron it needs.

Such a split leaves another molecule with an odd number of electrons, forming another free radical that reacts quickly by stealing an electron from a nearby molecule. When the attracted molecule loses its electrons, it also becomes a free radical and the chain reaction continues. When the body's natural defenses are exhausted, free radicals

Resveratrol in Foods

bilberries	peanuts (boiled or roasted)
blueberries	pistachios
cranberries	pomegranate juice
dark chocolate	raw cranberry juice
hops (an ingredient in beer)	red and purple grapes
lingonberries	red grape juice
peanut butter (preferably 100 percent natural)	red wine

Adapted from *The Longevity Factor* by Joseph Maroon.

continue to multiply and attack. Cells and whole organs can be damaged. While we are all subject to free radicals and the damage they cause, resveratrol and other antioxidants can counteract the effects of free radicals in our bodies. Because of this action, antioxidants like resveratrol are known as scavengers of free radicals. While this process may sound unpleasant, our health depends on it.

Antioxidants to the Rescue

We know that oxygen causes metals to rust or a cut apple to turn brown. Similarly, the human body "rusts" in its own way through a process called oxidation. Antioxidants block oxidation by donating an electron to an unstable molecule, thereby stabilizing it. With this unique ability, antioxidants stop the chain reaction of free radicals.

Resveratrol is an antioxidant. There are literally thousands of other antioxidants, which also are called phytochemicals. *Phyto* is the Greek word for plants, so this term translates as "plant chemicals" and is used to refer to any chemical that originates from a plant. Phytochemicals give fruits and vegetables their colors. Because plants with varying hues offer different health benefits, experts recommend including a variety of colorful foods in our diets—as many as three colors of fruits and vegetables with every meal. Several of the most protective phytochemicals are found abundantly in the skins and seeds of grapes.

Before the mid-1990s, antioxidant research focused on antioxidant vitamins, such as vitamins C and E, carotenoids, and minerals. The focus later switched to antioxidants from plants, like resveratrol. The scientific community began to recognize that phytochemicals protect against illnesses, including cancer, cardiovascular disease, diabetes, osteoporosis, and neurodegenerative diseases. In fact, antioxidants are known to combat the oxidative stress associated with nearly every degenerative disease. They also are associated with cell maintenance, DNA repair, and overall longevity. In addition, there is evidence that cancer patients who maintain adequate levels of antioxidants tolerate the high stress of chemotherapy better than those with low levels.

Certain phytochemicals offer greater antioxidant benefits than others. Scientists have devised several different ways to measure the

TABLE 2. Resveratrol content in wines and grape juice

Beverage	Total milligrams resveratrol per liter	Total milligrams resveratrol per 5-ounce glass
Red wines (global)	1.98–7.13	0.30–1.07
Red wines (Spanish)	1.92–12.59	0.29–1.89
Red grape juice (Spanish)	1.14–8.69	0.17–1.30
Rosé wines (Spanish)	0.43–3.52	0.06–0.53
White wines (Spanish)	0.05–1.80	0.01–0.27

Source: Linus Pauling Institute, Oregon State University, Micronutrient Information Center, http://lpi.oregonstate.edu/infocenter/phytochemicals/resveratrol.

antioxidant power of foods. For example, the FRAP (ferric-reducing ability of plasma) assay is one measure of a food's total antioxidant content. Using this method, researchers measured the antioxidant content of more than 3,100 foods, beverages, spices, herbs, and supplements, and published their findings in a 2010 edition of *Nutrition Journal*. The information in table 2, which shows the total antioxidant content of selected beverages, was drawn from their research. Red wine appears near the top of the list.

Earlier research, published in 2003 in the *Journal of Agricultural and Food Chemistry*, compared the total antioxidant capacities of black tea, cocoa, green tea, and red wine. The findings, gleaned through the use of different measures, or assays (ABTS and DPPH), showed cocoa as having the greatest antioxidant capacity, with red wine second, green tea third, and black tea fourth. Different techniques for measuring antioxidant content may yield somewhat different results, but despite slight changes in rank, red wine, cocoa, and tea are proven antioxidant powerhouses.

In 2010, United States Department of Agriculture (USDA) scientists published an extensive list of foods and their antioxidant activities. These researchers used a different system called ORAC values, or Oxygen Radical Absorption Capacity, to measure total antioxidant capacity in foods. Their results can be found on the USDA Agricultural Research Services website (www.ars.usda.gov). ORAC values now can be found on some product and supplement labels.

In 2004, other researchers had used ORAC values in determining results published in the *Journal of Agriculture and Food Chemistry*. Their measures of total antioxidant content in food are shown

TABLE 3. Beverages highest in antioxidants

Beverage	Antioxidant content*
Espresso, prepared	14.2
Coffee, prepared filtered and boiled	2.5
Red wine	2.5
Pomegranate juice	2.1
Green tea, prepared	1.5
Grape juice	1.2
Black tea, prepared	1.0
Prune juice	1.0
Cranberry juice	.92
Orange juice	.64
Tomato juice	.48
Cocoa with milk	.37
Apple juice	.27

*Antioxidant content is defined in mmol/100 g.
Source: Carlsen et al. *Nutrition Journal* 2010, 9:3.

in table 4 (see page 10). Interestingly, although we know red grapes and red wine to be very high in antioxidants, we see here that a few dozen foods ranked higher in overall antioxidant content. Red grapes and red wine still reign supreme in resveratrol content.

Polyphenols

One class of phytochemicals is the polyphenols, which are chemical compounds found in plants. Polyphenols are the most abundant antioxidants in our diets, present in quantities ten times greater than in vitamin C and 100 times greater than in vitamin E or carotenoids. Polyphenols are plentiful in fruits, vegetables, and plant-derived drinks, including red wine, coffee, fruit juices, and tea. They also are found in chocolate, cereal, and legumes. Today it is well established that polyphenols, obtained either through food or supplements, improve health status.

Polyphenols are classified according to their molecular composition and have more than one "phenol," or building block, per molecule. Polyphenols are further classified as flavonoids and nonflavonoids. Flavonoids (or bioflavonoids), one of the most nutritionally important classes of polyphenols, are aromatic and include many pigments. Fruits and vegetables that are rich in color contain greater amounts of flavonoids. In grapes the flavonoids are mostly anthocyanins. These powerful antioxidants give blue, purple, and red fruits and vegetables their color. The root of this word, *cyan*, means "blue."

Catechin and quercetin are among the most studied flavonoids. Catechins are abundant in green tea. Quercetin is found in red wine, apples, broccoli, grapes, and tea, and it is sometimes paired with resveratrol in supplements.

Enzymes

Without enzymes it would be impossible for us to absorb and process the nutrients in foods. Enzymes play a critical role in the transfer of resveratrol and other beneficial chemicals to our cells and are also indispensable to cellular health and growth. Resveratrol activates sirtuins, enzymes that play a key role in health and longevity. (See chapter 4, page 39.)

As catalysts, enzymes bring about chemical changes within the body. In fact, enzymes are known to create thousands of changes in the body. Enzymes play specific roles and are attracted only to their target substances. Any substance that an enzyme acts on is called the substrate. The name given to an enzyme is often, but not always, derived from the substrate by adding "ase" at the end. For example, lactose, a sugar found in milk, is changed by the enzyme lactase.

Enzyme activity can be affected by other molecules. Inhibitors are molecules that decrease enzyme activity; activators increase enzyme activity. Resveratrol is called a sirtuin activator.

Beyond Resveratrol:
The Power of Plants

Many research studies have proved what may seem like common sense: Plant-based diets protect us from illness. Beyond

TABLE 4. Foods highest in antioxidants

Rank	Food	Amount	Total antioxidant capacity*
1	small red beans, dried	1/2 cup	13,727
2	blueberries, wild	1 cup	13,427
3	red kidney beans, dried	1/2 cup	13,259
4	pinto beans, dried	1/2 cup	11,864
5	blueberries, cultivated	1 cup	9,019
6	cranberries, whole	1 cup	8,983
7	artichoke hearts, cooked	1 cup	7,904
8	blackberries	1 cup	7,701
9	prunes	1/2 cup	7,291
10	raspberries	1 cup	6,058
11	strawberries	1 cup	5,938
12	apple, red delicious	1 apple	5,900
13	apple, granny smith	1 apple	5,381
14	pecans	1 ounce	5,095
15	cherries, sweet	1 cup	4,873
16	plum, black	1 plum	4,844
17	potato, russet, cooked	1 potato	4,649
18	black beans, dried	1/2 cup	4,181
19	plum	1 plum	4,118
20	apple, gala	1 apple	3,903
21	walnuts	1 ounce	3,846
22	apple, golden delicious	1 apple	3,685

polyphenols, plant foods contain carotenoids, fiber, organic acids, sulfur compounds, phytosterols, and vitamins.

Studies involving food have become increasingly important. The period after World War II saw the development of processed foods high in fat and salt, and a fast-food culture that promoted convenient and inexpensive meals based on these poor-quality products. By the

TABLE 4. Continued

Rank	Food	Amount	Total antioxidant capacity*
23	apple, fuji	1 apple	3,578
24	dates, deglet noor	1/2 cup	3,467
25	avocado, hass	1 avocado	3,344
26	pear, green	1 pear	3,172
27	pear, red anjou	1 pear	2,943
28	hazelnuts	1 ounce	2,739
29	broccoli rabe, raw	1/5 bunch	2,621
30	navy beans, dried	1/2 cup	2,573
31	orange, navel	1 orange	2,540
32	figs, dried	1/2 cup	2,537
33	raisins	1/2 cup	2,490
34	cabbage, red, cooked,	1/2 cup	2,359
35	potato, red, raw	1 potato	2,339
36	potato, red, cooked	1 potato	2,294
37	pistachios	1 ounce	2,267
38	black-eyed peas, dried	1/2 cup	2,258
39	potato, white, raw	1 potato	2,257
40	dates, medjool	1/2 cup	2,124
41	asparagus, raw	1 cup	2,021
42	grapes, red	1 cup	2,016

*Total antioxidant capacity expressed in micromoles of Trolox, as used in the ORAC assay.

Source: USDA-ARS, Arkansas Children's Research Center, Little Rock, AR, 2004 data. *J Agric Food Chem*, 2004, 52:4026–37.

end of the twentieth century, the overconsumption of processed foods had created an epidemic of obesity. Along with increased weight came greater incidences of cancer, cardiac disease, and diabetes, serious health threats that are even more prevalent today.

What we choose to eat—and drink—is one critical factor in reversing this trend. Some antioxidant- and resveratrol-rich foods—like blueberries, chocolate, green tea, and peanuts—are nutrition superstars.

Bet on the Blue

Although they contain only about one-tenth the amount of resveratrol as red grapes, cultivated blueberries and wild blueberries in particular are loaded with anthocyanins and other beneficial plant chemicals. They have one of the highest ORAC values of all foods and rightfully take their place at or near the top of most experts' superfoods lists. Eating just one-half cup of blueberries per day helps lower blood pressure, promotes memory, and protects against cancer—more than any other any fruit. Because fresh blueberry season is regrettably short, frozen berries are an excellent alternative that can be found year-round. To make a healthful smoothie, blend frozen blueberries and a banana with nondairy milk, such as soymilk or almond milk. If you like, add a tablespoon of ground flaxseeds for omega-3 fatty acids.

Find Flavonol-Rich Chocolate

Natural cocoa, a source of resveratrol, has been cited as the highest source of antioxidants. Cocoa seeds are rich in a subclass of flavonoids called flavonols. Because of how they are processed, most commercial cocoas and chocolates retain few flavonols. So, you can't count vending-machine candy bars to be healthful. However, many experts agree that dark chocolate containing at least 70 percent cocoa content and no milk offers considerable health benefits.

Researchers like Norman Hollenberg are more discriminating. Hollenberg has researched the Kuni Indians, who live on islands off the Panama coast and drink at least five cups of natural cocoa with extremely high flavonol content every day. This population has very low blood pressure and a reduced frequency of cancer, diabetes, heart attack, and stroke. They also live longer than other Panamanians. Flavonol is the key. Hollenberg says if we don't know the flavonol content of our chocolate or cocoa, we can't evaluate its health benefits. Furthermore, he warns that judging chocolate by its color can be misleading. For example, dutch-process cocoa and chocolate may be very dark in color, but this alkalizing technique strips cocoa of its bitterness as well as most of its active flavonols.

Resveratrol: As Seen on TV

Although not especially easy to say or spell, "resveratrol" has become a common household term because of extensive media coverage. You may have seen some of the following television shows that have featured stories about resveratrol:

- In 1991, the television news program *60 Minutes* aired a segment about the French paradox and red wine's ability to reduce heart disease. Afterward, consumption of red wine increased 44 percent, and some wineries even lobbied for the right to label their wines as "health food." In 2009, *60 Minutes* once again featured red wine and resveratrol. By then, scientists had discovered that significant doses of resveratrol triggered a longevity gene, potentially promising us an additional decade or two of healthy old age. Find the video *Wine Rx* at www.cbsnews.com.

- In April 2008, Barbara Walters interviewed researcher David Sinclair about resveratrol and the longevity gene. Activating it can not only extend life but also help us avoid diseases like cancer, heart disease, and even osteoporosis. Find the video *Drink Red Wine and Live Longer* at www.abcnews.com.

- In 2009, separate segments on Oprah Winfrey's show featured physician Mehmet Oz discussing the benefits of resveratrol and actor Michael J. Fox speaking about resveratrol's potential to protect against Parkinson's disease. (See www.Oprah.com.) Oz, medical director, Integrative Medicine Program, NewYork-Presbyterian Hospital/Columbia University Medical Center, has since launched his own television program, *The Dr. Oz Show*, and periodically discusses resveratrol.

Note: While these celebrities have reported on resveratrol, they do not represent or endorse any resveratrol supplement or manufacturer. Although they are frequently featured in ads for resveratrol supplements, they have taken legal action against manufacturers that unlawfully use their names and likenesses. Find information about choosing a resveratrol supplement in chapter 3.

Drink Lots of Green

The health benefits of green tea, which is rich in catechins, are similar to those of resveratrol and red wine. Green tea is a strong antioxidant with antiaging effects. It also interferes with cancer development and growth. In terms of heart health, it reduces clotting and high blood pressure and elevates high-density lipoprotein (HDL), or "good," cholesterol, leading to fewer heart attacks. In addition, green tea can accel

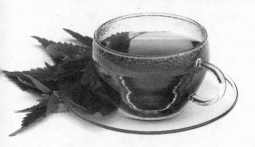

erate weight loss. Benefits from green tea are optimal when you drink three to ten cups daily, which is common in some cultures. To boost the benefits of drinking green tea, squeeze in a little lemon juice, which will enhance your ability to absorb the tea's beneficial catechins.

Go a Little Nuts

Technically, peanuts aren't nuts (they are legumes), but they offer some of the same health benefits as tree nuts, which, when eaten frequently in small quantities, can reduce the risk of heart disease by more than half. Several factors in peanuts may contribute to this healthful effect. Peanuts, which contain resveratrol, also are an excellent source of vitamin E and fiber and have relatively high amounts of copper, folic acid, magnesium, manganese, niacin, phosphorus, thiamin, and zinc. In addition, they are high in plant protein and contain primarily mono

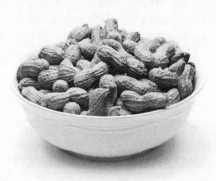

unsaturated and polyunsaturated fat. Some people avoid peanuts because of their high caloric value. However, studies show that regular peanut eaters have a lower body mass index (BMI) than people who don't eat peanuts. Snackers typically are satisfied after eating only a small amount of peanuts, and this helps offset the nut's concentrated calories.

A History of Healing

In addition to being a source of food, plants have been valued throughout history for their medicinal qualities. Traditional medicine (also known as alternative or complementary medicine), which is based on plants and herbs, has been used for thousands of years in cultures around the world. According to the World Health Orga nization, in some Asian and African countries up to 80 percent of the population still depend on traditional medicine for their primary health care. In countries such as the United States, 70 to 80 percent of the population have used some form of alternative treatment, like herbal medicine.

Modern medicine also relies on plants. Early drugs used in Western medicine were plant-derived extracts. About 25 percent of prescription drugs are derived from plants. An example is the drug paclitaxel, which was developed from the Pacific yew tree and is used to treat lung, breast, and ovarian cancer. Still, only a fraction of plant species have been tested to see whether they have medicinal potential. Different parts of each plant (flower, leaf, root) can have different effects.

Today, anthropologists and other scientists investigate other cultures to determine what plants they use for healing. This field of ethnobotany has introduced new plants for pharmaceutical research.

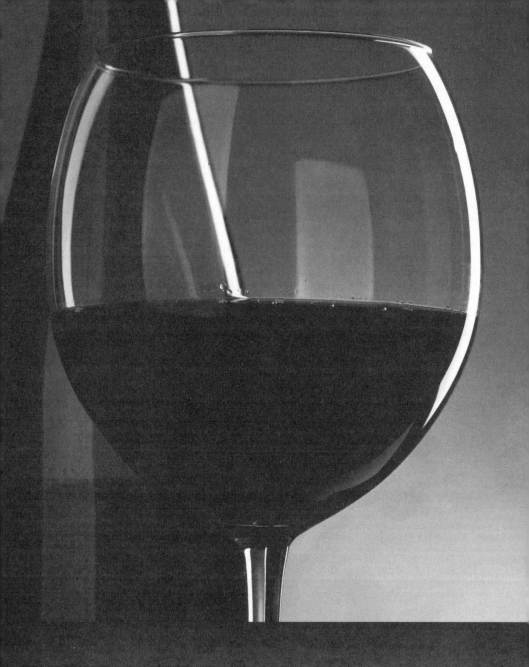

Just love your brother and drink a good glass of red wine every day.

Advice from Antonio Todde,
Once the world's oldest man, who lived to age 112

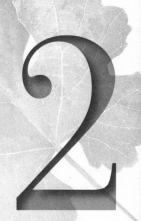

Red Wine and Health

enturies ago, Greek hosts wished guests good health when raising a glass of wine. This action had a slightly dark side then: By taking the first sip, the host satisfied his guests that the wine was safe to drink. Now a friendly tradition, salutes to health and long life ring out over wineglasses worldwide.

Could the Greeks—in fact, could any of us—have dreamed that wine, good health, and long life would someday be connected in very scientific terms? Today, research shows us that they are, with resveratrol and other powerful phytochemicals at the core.

Researchers have looked at what we drink *and* eat to find health-promoting relationships. Red wine has featured prominently in this quest. The wine-growing regions of France—along with regions on the Mediterranean coast, including Greece, Crete, southern Italy, and Spain—have received particular attention. The consumption of red wine, along with an abundance of fresh fruits and vegetables, has granted denizens of these regions exceptional health and longevity.

The French Paradox

In the early 1800s, an Irish physician noted that despite their high-fat diet, the French were, in general, a healthy population. This puzzling contradiction was noted again about twenty years ago when epidemiologists observed that the French, while eating a diet high in saturated fats, had the lowest incidence of heart disease in

Europe. In 1991, a scientist at France's Bordeaux University used the term "French paradox" to describe this phenomenon. That same year, a news story about the French paradox aired on the television show *60 Minutes*. The term quickly caught on in the media and was readily adopted into our language.

Recognition of the French paradox initiated research around the world. A 1992 study reported in the British journal *The Lancet* provided an interesting perspective: consumption of wine and alcohol equivalent to the intake in France (20 to 30 grams daily) reduced the risk of coronary artery disease by at least 40 percent. In the face of such promising findings, researchers focused on antioxidants in red wine in hopes of discovering which specific compounds had the most health-promoting properties.

The Mediterranean Diet

In June 1995, Walter Willett, of the Harvard School of Public Health, and other epidemiologists, from the University of Minnesota School of Public Health, put the Mediterranean diet on the map. Intrigued by the low rates of chronic disease among people living in this region, these scientists reviewed epidemiologic evidence to identify the contributing dietary factors. The resulting articles in the *American Journal of Clinical Nutrition* sharpened science's focus on the Mediterranean diet, which is still described as a model diet today.

In reviewing the available research, Willett and his colleagues concluded that the following factors contributed to the excellent health and long life expectancies of Mediterranean populations:

- high consumption of fruit, vegetables, and whole grains
- moderate intake of alcohol
- low consumption of animal products and saturated and hydrogenated fats

Reviewers noted that this eating pattern was typical of Crete, much of the rest of Greece, and southern Italy in the early 1960s. That is when people in these regions experienced the world's greatest life expectancy and the lowest rates of coronary artery disease, certain cancers, and other diet-related chronic diseases. Back then, low rates of obesity were the result of excellent diets in combination with regular physical activity, such as field or kitchen work.

Recent research about the Mediterranean diet confirms its viability today. A 2007 article in the *Archives of Internal Medicine* examined the effects of this diet on a large U.S. population. This article reported the results of the National Institutes of Health–AARP Diet and Health Study, which included more than 380,000 subjects (214,284 men and 166,012 women), members of the American Association of Retired Persons who resided in six states. The Mediterranean diet as defined by this study included vegetables, legumes, fruits, nuts, whole grains, fish, monounsaturated fat, alcohol, and some meat. The result? This eating style was associated with reduced mortality (proportion of deaths to population) from all causes, as well as reduced mortality from cardiovascular disease and cancer. Specific health benefits associated with the diet included reduced chronic inflammation, low concentrations of oxidized LDL ("bad") cholesterol, and a low omega-6 to omega-3 fatty acid ratio, which potentially prevents and slows cancer.

Similar results were reported in a study published in the *British Medical Journal* in 2009. Researchers followed more than twenty-three thousand Greek men and women for more than eight years to see how the Mediterranean diet affected mortality. Results showed that some components of the Mediterranean diet, particularly high vegetable consumption and low meat consumption, were associated

A Look at Lifestyle

When we look at the greater cultural context, we can identify potential reasons beyond food and drink that contribute to the health of Mediterranean and French people. For example, the design of what we now call the Mediterranean diet was based on eating patterns prevalent in the early 1960s, a time when this population largely relied on heavy physical activity for their livelihoods. Theirs also was a place and time as yet unaffected by many modern stressors. Similarly, perhaps the French paradox can be explained in part by this culture's *joie de vivre* and tradition of dining with companions. Social connections improve digestion and overall health. As we make choices about our own health, it's important to consider lifestyle aspects in addition to what we eat or drink.

with a lower risk of mortality than other diet components. High consumption of fruits, nuts, and legumes, along with moderate alcohol intake, also were associated with lower mortality risk.

Clearly the Mediterranean diet and other plant-based diets offer timeless benefits. Beyond the long-acknowledged role this diet can play in preventing heart disease, cancer, and chronic disease, the Mediterranean diet may also reduce the risk of cognitive decline as we age. According to study results released in May 2010 by researchers with the Chicago Health and Aging Project, of four thousand participants age sixty-five and older, those who ranked highest in terms of following a Mediterranean-type diet were more protected from cognitive decline. Researchers recommended that older adults eat more olive oil, legumes, nuts, and seeds to improve recall times and other cognitive skills.

All Wines Are Not Created Equal

Great variations are found when the resveratrol content of red wines is compared. Factors that affect the amount of resveratrol in a bottle of wine include how the wine is processed, the type of grape and vintage, and climatic characteristics in the growing region. Resveratrol concentrations are generally higher in red wines made from grapes grown in cooler regions or other areas with extreme weather. This makes sense when we consider resveratrol's role in protecting plants from enemies like cold and fungal infection.

Want to get more resveratrol from your wine? Here are some tips:

- Uncork a variety high in resveratrol content. North American wines made from the muscadine grape may have a higher resveratrol content than wine made from European grapes. Of these, pinot noir, merlot, and cabernet sauvignon are among those thought to have the highest levels (see table 5, page 21).

- Compare resveratrol content by reading labels. The U.S. government now allows wine producers to provide this information on bottles. Amounts greater than 10 micromoles per liter are considered high.

- Go organic. Grapevines that are not protected by commercial chemicals must protect themselves. Unprotected grapes are likely

TABLE 5. Concentrations of resveratrol in wine varietals

Wine varietal	Country of origin	Resveratrol concentration*
Red**	Brazil	18 mg/L
Pinot noir	Australia	13.4 mg/L
Pinot noir	California	5.5 mg/L
Pinot noir	Spain	5.1 mg/L
Red**	Switzerland	5.0–12.3 mg/L
Rhone Valley reds	France	3.6 mg/L
Bordeaux reds	France	3.9 mg/L
Cabernet sauvignon	Australia	1.7 mg/L
Cabernet sauvignon	California	0.9 mg/L
Red grape juice	n/a	0.5 mg/L

*Results reported in milligrams per liter.

**Varietal not stated.

Source: Opie, L. and S. Lecour. 2007. "The Red Wine Hypothesis: From Concepts to Protective Signalling Molecules." *European Heart Journal* 28: 1688.

to produce much greater amounts of resveratrol, ultimately resulting in higher levels in organic wines as well.

- Select unfiltered wines and grape juice, which are likely to contain more resveratrol and other healthful polyphenols than filtered products.

- Savor your wine slowly, allowing it to linger in your mouth before swallowing. Some researchers propose that the mouth's mucous membranes can absorb more resveratrol than the gut, resulting in far greater blood levels of resveratrol.

- Watch for new trends on the market. For example, resveratrol-enhanced wines are now becoming available.

Red Wine versus Other Types of Alcohol

When it comes to red wine, drinking moderate amounts has long been considered good for our hearts and may also increase our longevity. The polyphenols in red wine, such as flavonoids and resveratrol, often get the credit for these health advantages. Red

How Much Wine Is Healthful?

The well-known health benefits of red wine should not be used as an excuse for drinking too much. Medical experts recommend no more than two drinks per day for men and one drink per day for women. When it comes to wine, one glass is typically described as five ounces. Many people, however, drink more than that in one serving.

You can test your own habits by pouring wine in a measuring cup until it reaches about one-half cup. Then pour the wine from the measuring cup into the wineglass you usually use. Match that level when pouring yourself a glass of wine in the future.

More wine does not equal more health benefits. In fact, drinking three or more glasses a day can do your heart more harm than good, increasing your blood pressure and your risk of heart disease and stroke. Plus, alcohol is high in calories and can contribute to weight gain and associated illnesses. One five-ounce glass of red wine has around 120 calories.

wine's superiority over other types of alcohol, however, has been the subject of considerable controversy.

Some researchers maintain that red wine confers more health advantages than other types of alcohol. Others say that alcohol itself is the source of health benefits, contending that red wine provides no more benefits than white wine, beer, or hard liquor. A reasonable explanation for this disparity is that lifestyle factors beyond red wine or alcohol use—such as diet, exercise, or socioeconomic status—affect health outcomes as well as research results. The bottom line seems to be that, when consumed sensibly in moderation, all types of alcohol offer potential health benefits. Red wine, however, seems to provide a particular advantage. Here is some of the research on this matter.

In a 1993 study published in the British medical journal *The Lancet*, researchers compared the effects of alcohol versus the polyphenols in red wine. They reported that the nonalcoholic components of red wine have potent antioxidant properties toward LDL ("bad") cholesterol. (LDL particles appear to be harmless until they are oxidized in the blood vessels by free radicals.) Furthermore, the research showed that even when it was diluted one thousandfold, the wine showed significantly more antioxidant activity than alpha-tocopherol, a form of vitamin E that, at the time, was considered to be one of the most powerful antioxidants.

A 1997 study published in the *American Journal of Cardiology* concluded that in the presence of red wine or grape juice, LDL was significantly resistant to oxidation. This effect was not seen in alcohol (ethanol) alone, nor in nonflavonoid phenolic compounds.

One well-known study published in the December 11, 1997, edition of the *New England Journal of Medicine* weighed the pros and the cons of alcohol use but did not distinguish the types of alcohol used by study participants. This research showed that people of middle age or older who consumed moderate amounts of alcohol had a slightly reduced risk of mortality and lower death rates from coronary artery disease and stroke. The overall death rate was lowest among men and women who reported having about one drink daily. On the other hand, men and women who drank regularly, when compared with nondrinkers, had higher death rates from injuries, violence, suicide, poisoning, cirrhosis, certain cancers, and possibly hemorrhagic stroke.

A 2005 summary of research on red wine and alcohol appeared in the American Heart Association's journal *Circulation*. Reviewers looked at both epidemiological study results (of human populations) and biological studies that focused on molecular components. When the results of fifty-two epidemiological studies were combined, they showed that the risk of coronary artery disease decreased by about 20 percent in people who drank up to two alcoholic drinks per day. Other studies showed even greater percentages. Results from the Health Professionals Follow-Up Study, in which 38,077 male health professionals who were free of cardiovascular disease were observed for twelve years, suggested that drinking one to two alcoholic drinks per day, three to four days per week, decreased the risk of heart attack by as much as 32 percent.

Reviewers then evaluated claims that red wine confers additional benefits. The Copenhagen City Heart Study, in which 13,285 men and women were observed for twelve years, suggested that those who drank wine had half the risk of dying from coronary artery disease or stroke as those who never drank wine. Those who drank beer or hard liquor did not experience this benefit. Furthermore, an analysis of thirteen studies involving 209,418 participants showed a 32 percent reduced risk of atherosclerotic disease for red-wine drinkers and a 22 percent reduction for beer drinkers.

In 2007, an extensive review printed in the *European Heart Journal* evaluated the results of 136 studies about red wine and alcohol.

These reviewers concluded that red wine has beneficial effects "beyond alcohol," meaning that ethanol alone does not promote heart health or longer life to the same extent as red wine. However, they confirmed findings that modest alcohol intake from any source (versus not drinking at all or drinking heavily) reduces cardiovascular risk and overall mortality.

The authors of this review concluded that red wine is the drink of choice for those seeking the greatest health benefits from alcohol. They went on to describe the most convincing data as coming from human studies that measured the benefits of dealcoholized wine. These studies showed that even without the alcohol this beverage provided protective cardiovascular effects, which the authors attributed to polyphenols. Resveratrol, they noted, remains the most powerful of the polyphenols and one of the most likely to give biological protection.

Some researchers contend that components other than resveratrol are responsible for the good health bestowed on red-wine drinkers. Roger Corder, a London researcher and author of *The Red Wine Diet*, argues that substances called procyanidins are the source of red wine's many health benefits. Corder says these condensed tannins protect red-wine drinkers from heart disease, diabetes, and dementia. Healthful procyanidins also can be found in apples, berries, dark chocolate, and tea.

As the red-wine debate continues, researchers may embrace the probability that no single component confers all the benefits, but rather that several components contribute in different ways. For example, both resveratrol and procyanidins are beneficial ingredients in red wine. Furthermore, the mostly unexplored synergy between phytochemicals and alcohol may someday reveal the true health powers of red wine.

Alcohol and Heart Health

The preceding information about red wine and other types of alcohol focuses on the cardioprotective role they play. Although moderate use of alcohol has long been associated with heart health, the American Heart Association warns that more than two drinks per day for men and one for women can increase such dangers as alcoholism, high blood pressure, obesity, stroke, suicides, accidents, and breast cancer. Furthermore, the American Heart Association warns nondrinkers *not* to start drinking alcohol in hopes of improving their health. Alcohol can be a double-edged sword, especially when used in excess.

Alcohol and Cancer

Like the American Heart Association, the American Cancer Society recommends no more than two drinks per day for men and one for women. Years of research have established a clear relationship between alcohol use and some cancers, including breast, colon, esophagus, liver, mouth, rectum, throat, and voice box.

Early resveratrol research provided good news for heart health but spurred concerns that, as a phytoestrogen, resveratrol could stimulate growth of breast cancer cells. For years, women were cautioned about wine's possible link to breast cancer.

In December 2002, results from a large study performed by the American Cancer Society underscored the dangerous association between alcohol use and fatal breast cancer. Researchers found that, in comparison to nondrinkers, postmenopausal women who consumed one drink a day had a 30 percent greater chance of dying from breast cancer. The type of alcohol didn't seem to be a factor.

The March 4, 2009, edition of the *Journal of the National Cancer Institute* reported even more sobering findings about women's cancer risk and alcohol. In the Million Women Study, University of Oxford scientists tracked alcohol use and cancer in nearly 1.3 million middle-aged women in the United Kingdom (UK). Researchers concluded that, each year in the UK, alcohol accounted for about 22 percent of liver cancers, 11 percent of breast cancers, 9 percent of rectal cancers, and 25 percent of cancers of the esophagus, oral cavity, throat, and voice box. Cancer risk increased with the number of drinks a woman consumed, regardless of what kind of alcohol she drank. An editorial that accompanied these findings concluded that, from the standpoint of cancer risk, no level of alcohol consumption could be considered safe.

Alcohol and Older Adults

According to the National Institute on Aging, older adults may face more risks from drinking alcohol. Certain health problems

Wine Alert for Vegetarians and Vegans

Although you might not suspect that animal products would be used in producing wine and other alcohols, such items can be used in "fining," a process that makes these beverages clear. Many wines undergo some degree of fining with agents such as gelatin, isinglass (obtained from the swim bladders of fish), egg white, or other products. To avoid these, choose wines that have not been fined, or contact the winemaker to learn how your favorite wine is fined.

in older adults—including stroke, high blood pressure, memory loss, and mood disorders—may be made worse with alcohol use.

Research in this area has shown that alcohol's effect on older adults may rely greatly on their health status. Men and women over age fifty who are in good to excellent health can experience health benefits when they drink light to moderate amounts of alcohol, according to the results of a study published in the *American Journal of Epidemiology* in 2009. By analyzing self-reported data from 4,200 study participants, researchers concluded that light to moderate drinkers, compared to heavy drinkers or nondrinkers, reduced their risks of becoming disabled or dying in the following five years by 23 percent. Researchers emphasized that reduced risks applied only to those who were already in good health; those who reported being only in fair or in poor health gained no benefits from drinking alcohol.

Alternatives to Red Wine

If you are unable to drink red wine or simply choose not to, you can still enjoy the benefits of resveratrol from other sources. Here are some tips:

- Eat foods such as red and purple grapes and berries, peanuts, dark chocolate, and other resveratrol-rich foods that are listed in the box on page 5. Note that conventionally grown table grapes aren't likely to contain much resveratrol; homegrown and organic grapes can have significantly more.

- Drink grape juice. Resveratrol is found in 100 percent grape juice, especially in juice made from dark purple concord grapes. Organic and unfiltered juices are likely to contain the most resveratrol. In general, grape juice contains about half the amount of flavonoids by volume as red wine.

- Take a supplement. (See chapter 3, page 29.)

- Evaluate new resveratrol products carefully. Some processed foods claim to provide a resveratrol punch. New but untested products include resveratrol juice, a resveratrol nutrition bar, and a resveratrol energy shot. Resveratrol gum and lozenges reportedly are on the way.

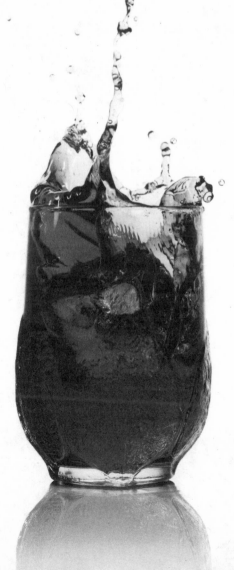

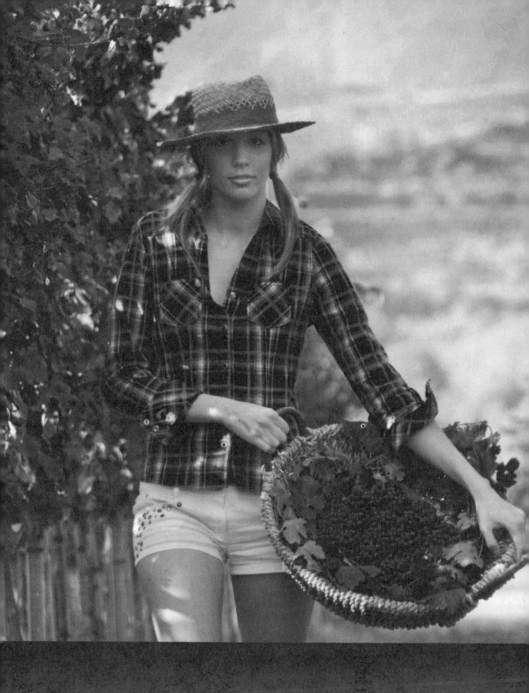

The first wealth is health.

Ralph Waldo Emerson

Resveratrol Supplements

A daily dietary supplement can provide a far greater amount of resveratrol than a glass or two of red wine—or even many, many bottles of red wine, each of which typically contains only one to three milligrams of resveratrol. In fact, you would have to drink 750 to 1,500 bottles of wine *per day* to get amounts of resveratrol equal to those used in some widely publicized animal research studies.

Using supplements is a realistic and affordable option. Some brands are more costly, but they may not be superior. A high-quality resveratrol supplement can cost as little as $25 to $30 per month, which many people consider to be a sound investment in their health. According to survey results released in 2010 by ConsumerLab, an independent testing laboratory, 19.4 percent of survey respondents reported using resveratrol, and sales had increased 66 percent in only one year.

One-quarter of U.S. adults use herbal supplements at least occasionally, and more than half use vitamin supplements regularly. Overall, annual supplement sales are about $25 billion a year. Despite their popularity, dietary supplements are not reviewed or regulated like prescription drugs. That is why we see language like this on supplement labels and in ads: "This statement has not been evaluated by the Food and Drug Administration (FDA). This product is not intended to diagnose, treat, cure, or prevent any disease." The FDA only becomes involved when there are harmful reports about certain supplements.

Given the lack of regulation and such sweeping disclaimers, disreputable manufacturers can make any claims they want to about their products without substantiating them. The situation has been likened to Dodge City, uncontrolled and lawless. Unless you have done your homework, selecting a resveratrol supplement can feel like shooting in the dark.

Given the buzz about resveratrol in the past decade, supplement manufacturers have jumped at the chance to capitalize on resveratrol's potential. More and more products appear on the market, and our many options can leave us bewildered in the supplement aisle or when we shop online. The big question is this: If you decide to go the supplement route, how can you have confidence in the product you buy?

There are several reputable brands of supplemental resveratrol, and the tips that follow will help you make an educated choice. These tips can be helpful when choosing nutritional supplements in general. One of your best options is to find out what independent testing labs have to say about specific brands of supplements. (See box, page 31.)

Buyer Beware

In a surprising number of cases, when supplements are tested, they are found to lack active ingredients in the amounts advertised. For example, when ConsumerLab first tested one brand of resveratrol supplement, they found that, contrary to claims on the label, resveratrol represented only a tiny fraction of the total blended content. The manufacturer updated the label simply by removing any reference to the amount of resveratrol in its product, yet there is nothing illegal about the labeling for this product. A physician who has written a book about resveratrol is a paid spokesman for this supplement manufacturer. Many supplement manufacturers hire professional spokespeople, a fact that underscores the importance of researching your sources when making a decision as important as which supplement to take.

One critical step in finding a supplement that works for you is reading labels. There are different types of resveratrol. The one typically used in supplements is called *trans*-resveratrol. This is the form that has been shown to affect aging in mice. Some supplement labels

Researching Brands of Resveratrol

Independent, third-party testing can help answer our critical questions about resveratrol and other supplements. One resource is ConsumerLab, an independent laboratory that has tested more than two thousand supplements made by more than three hundred manufacturers. In their tests, one in four supplements has been found to have quality problems.

ConsumerLab provides brand-specific resveratrol ratings for a fee. Its current resveratrol report evaluates fifteen brands. At consumerlab.com, you can buy the resveratrol report for $12, or you can buy an annual subscription that provides access to reports about multiple supplements.

ConsumerLab answers the following question when evaluating resveratrol supplements:

- Does the supplement contain resveratrol as listed on the label, in the declared potency and amounts?
- Does the supplement contain impurities, such as lead or cadmium, which can occur in plant-based supplements?
- Will the supplement break down and release into the body properly?
- What is the supplement cost per 100 milligrams of resveratrol?

Government resources also provide helpful information for free. The National Library of Medicine Supplement Labels Database, for example, contains fifteen resveratrol entries. Overall, the database includes information about label ingredients in more than four thousand selected brands of dietary supplements. Find the database at http://dietarysupplements.nlm.nih.gov/dietary. An additional government resource about dietary supplements can be found at http://ods.od.nih.gov, the website of the National Institutes of Health Office of Dietary Supplements.

simply describe the contents as *trans*-resveratrol. Most, however, name specific ingredients in the Supplement Facts box. The active ingredient in most resveratrol supplements is Japanese knotweed, which may be listed on the label as *Polygonum cuspidatum*, giant knotweed, or *hu zhang*. Japanese knotweed is an affordable commercial source of resveratrol that is thought to be as effective as grapes, a more expensive source. Some resveratrol supplements are augmented with grape skin, grapeseed, or red-wine extracts.

Choose a supplement that includes the word "resveratrol" in the name. ConsumerLab's president, Todd Cooperman, warns that 300 milligrams of a "red-wine complex" or "proprietary formula" is not the same as 300 milligrams of resveratrol itself. In fact, supplements with the term "red wine" in the name contain little wine. And supplements with the words "grape skin" in the name may claim to contain resveratrol but may not say how much. Grapeseed extract is a commercial formulation that does not contain resveratrol.

Supplements that pair resveratrol with quercetin appear to boost the resveratrol's effectiveness. To elevate both health claims and sales, manufacturers of resveratrol supplements may also feature substances such as acai, calcium, green tea, pomegranate, and vitamin C. When a specific synergy with resveratrol has not been established, as is the case with quercetin, choosing a single-ingredient supplement over one with multiple ingredients can be a smart move. For one thing, such a choice can reduce your consumption of potential contaminants and other undesirable or unwanted ingredients.

Some unwanted ingredients in supplements are fillers, binders, and common allergens. These typically are listed underneath the Supplement Facts box on labels, making it easy for consumers to avoid them by choosing an alternative product. Unfortunately, supplements may also contain dangerous components, such as heavy metals and other toxins. This information, of course, will not appear on the packaging. We must rely on independent reviews and reputable news outlets to reveal such harmful ingredients.

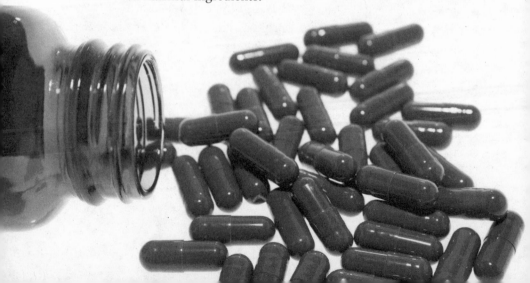

When shopping for resveratrol supplements, one strategy is to compare ingredients and disqualify supplements that contain items you want to avoid. For instance, vegetarians and vegans purchase supplements made without gelatin or other animal ingredients. To ensure that your supplement contains no animal ingredients, look for a logo or seal that indicates the product has been certified. For example, the American Vegetarian Association certifies that certain supplements are vegan.

Some experts recommend choosing a capsule that is produced and packaged in an oxygen-free environment to prevent degradation. Over time, more manufacturers are taking these precautions and say so on supplement labels and in marketing materials. One study funded by a supplement manufacturer contested this advice, concluding that resveratrol is more stable and less sensitive to oxidation than previously thought.

And finally, avoid imported supplements as a rule. An increasing number have been found to not only include undesirable fillers but also to be spiked with illegal drugs.

Dosage Dilemma

Just as there is no government regulation of resveratrol supplements, there also is no recommended dosage. Resveratrol supplements typically contain up to 500 milligrams per capsule; the amount is determined solely by the manufacturer. Researchers caution that scientific study in humans must occur before usage and dosage recommendations can be made.

That said, several researchers and physicians have discussed the amounts of resveratrol that they take or recommend to their patients:

- The *New York Times* reported that David Sinclair, a prominent resveratrol researcher who admits taking high doses of resveratrol, bases his dose on body weight. He follows the formula of 5 milligrams of resveratrol per kilogram (about 2.2 pounds) of body weight.
- In his book *The Longevity Factor*, physician and author Joseph Maroon says he takes 250 to 500 milligrams of resveratrol per day.
- Physician Mehmet Oz, host of *The Dr. Oz Show*, has discussed resveratrol on his program. In one episode, he described a typical supplement dose as 500 milligrams per day.

- In the book *Fantastic Voyage*, authors Ray Kurzweil and physician Terry Grossman recommend 400 milligrams of resveratrol daily.

Note that some supplement manufacturers may not list resveratrol content in milligrams but may instead use micrograms (mcg or μg). One thousand micrograms is equivalent to one milligram, so content given in micrograms may look like a large amount when it really is not.

Few human studies have been designed to determine safe dosages. A small study of ten people who took single doses of up to 5 grams of resveratrol—an amount many times greater than that contained in any single supplement—showed no serious adverse effects. Laboratory research using animal species have not raised safety concerns.

Even though there are unanswered questions about resveratrol supplementation, the potential benefits appear to outweigh the risks. Over time, as results of clinical trials are published, we will have more information to guide us. Until more is known, some people may prefer to sip a glass of red wine with dinner, which represents little risk for those who tolerate alcohol well and for women who are not pregnant.

Common-Sense Precautions

Despite the general safety profile of resveratrol, it's smart to take some precautions before using it in supplement form. Talk to your doctor about your interest. Even if she is not familiar with resveratrol supplements or supplements in general, she may be helpful in discussing your medical conditions and any that warrant consideration before using supplements. Here are some examples:

- Resveratrol supplements are not recommended for people with high blood pressure or heart failure.
- Taking resveratrol along with herbs or medications intended to thin the blood (anticoagulants) may increase the risk of bleeding.
- Pregnant women, nursing women, and women with a history of breast, uterine, or ovarian cancers should avoid resveratrol supplements, as they may affect estrogen activity.
- Growing children should not be given resveratrol supplements.

Research has shown that nutritional supplementation, particularly with antioxidants, can help improve health status and increase longevity. That does not mean that supplements can replace a healthful diet rich in fruits and vegetables. Rather, they are an effective complement.

Go Online at Your Own Risk

Knowledge provides a powerful advantage in maintaining your health, and it's wise to do your own research before buying a nutritional supplement. However, when you look for resveratrol information on the internet, it's critical to consider the source. Information provided by manufacturers or others who can profit from supplement sales deserves particular scrutiny. Unfortunately, the internet makes it easy for companies to disguise themselves, their advertising, and their real objectives.

Some supplement companies go to great lengths to make their online information look like it's coming from independent sources. This effort is called "disguised advertising," a marketing technique that has been used in promoting resveratrol supplements. For example, consumer advocacy organizations and attorney generals in multiple states have investigated a manufacturer that posted phony television news websites to promote its brand of supplements. These deceptive sites are convincing because they appear to be legitimate local news outlets.

Here are some tips for identifying questionable online information and marketing gimmicks:

- Follow the money. Sites, articles, or disguised ads that recommend or describe one superior resveratrol supplement or link to information about one particular brand may have been created by the manufacturer. A seemingly objective "article" may conclude with a recommendation or a link to a retail site. Even peer-reviewed articles in medical journals should be considered carefully because some research is funded by supplement manufacturers.

- Avoid promises of "free samples." Sites that require your credit card information to cover shipping and handling fees for free samples may be hiding important details in the fine print. Your card may be charged monthly for regular shipments of resveratrol unless you cancel within a specific time frame, such as ten

Resveratrol for Rover

People who buy resveratrol supplements for themselves can now do the same for their canine or feline companions. The capsules are said to contain anti-inflammatory and anticancer properties; to promote many advantages, including cardiovascular health; and to keep dogs and cats from acting old before their time. However, as is the case for humans, we must await solid research that supports such claims.

days, after requesting or receiving your sample. This practice has surprised and angered thousands of resveratrol buyers, many of whom never recovered their losses. Online resources, such as ComplaintsBoard.com and the Better Business Bureau (www.bbb.org), reveal consumer complaints and F ratings associated with disreputable companies that engage in these misleading practices.

- Be wary of false celebrity endorsements. It seems you can't go online these days without seeing resveratrol ads that feature television celebrities, such as Mehmet Oz of *The Dr. Oz Show*, Barbara Walters, and Oprah Winfrey. While these individuals have reported news about resveratrol on television, none endorses any particular brand. In fact, they have released disclaimers through their producers and networks and have taken legal action against companies that unlawfully use their names and images to promote supplements. References to reports from *60 Minutes* about resveratrol and researcher David Sinclair's work also appear frequently in online ads that could trick readers into assuming there is an endorsement.

- Pass on pop-ups. When it comes to supplement sales, disreputable companies have used this online device to draw attention to their products.

To find reliable online information about resveratrol, concentrate on well-known news websites. For example, the *New York Times* and science reporter Nicholas Wade have provided comprehensive coverage of resveratrol for years. Other publications, such as *Fortune*, *Newsweek*, and *Time*, also have featured articles about resveratrol. Going to these news websites and searching for the term "resveratrol" will produce multiple hits.

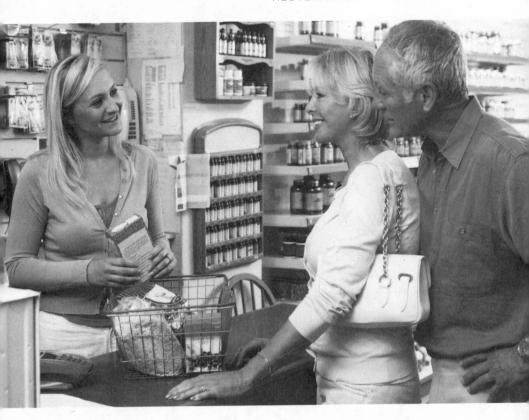

Note, however, that some reputable brands of resveratrol are dis-tributed via respected online retailers or directly from manufacturers' websites. If you prefer, you may buy your supplements in a store you know and trust. Ideally, talk to the pharmacist or a knowledgeable staff member about available brands.

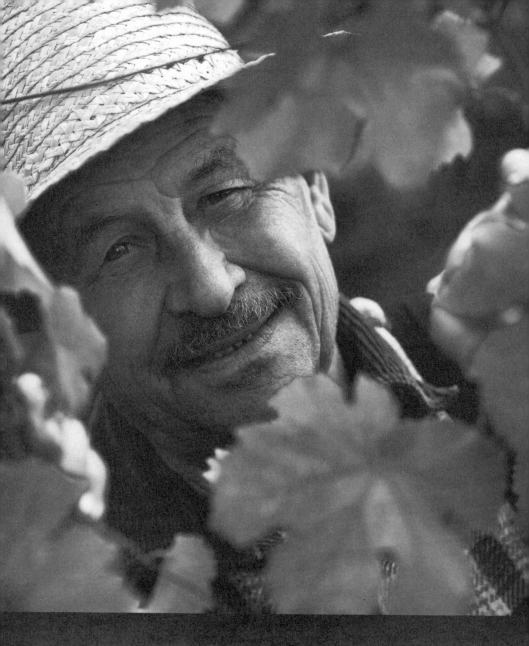

*Getting old is a fascinating thing.
The older you get, the older you
want to get.*

Keith Richards of the *Rolling Stones*

The New Fountain of Youth

ive centuries ago, Spanish explorer Juan Ponce de León searched for the legendary Fountain of Youth, which reputedly restores youth to anyone who is fortunate enough to drink from it. A variation of this quest continues today in science labs around the world. Scientists are not only seeking cures for the diseases associated with aging; they are also looking for ways to increase our longevity.

You may ask: How long do I want to live if being old means having diseases like Alzheimer's, cancer, diabetes, heart disease, and stroke? Of course, anyone who equates old age with illness and disability will dread growing old. The goal of longevity research is to prolong a healthy life so that people can enjoy more fulfilling and productive years.

Science has asked diverse questions about how and why we age. Is it possible that our bodies simply begin to wear out after our reproductive years have passed? This argument is logical from an evolutionary viewpoint, and it has prevailed among aging theories. Still, this hypothesis has had plenty of competition: over time, there have been more than three hundred theories on aging.

One theory proposes that aging is the simultaneous occurrence of many late-onset diseases; another states that aging is purely the result of our genetic programming. Other theories have prompted researchers to ask if aging is controlled by our metabolic rates, immune systems, or environments. New aging research has focused on aging at the cellular level and has revealed specific genes that are involved in the aging process. This is promising news, provided we can learn how to control the genes associated with aging.

Several aging theories are linked to resveratrol. The free radical theory hypothesizes that free radicals are responsible for age-related damage to our cells and tissues. As described in chapter 1, resveratrol is a powerful antioxidant that can reduce oxidative damage and preserve cellular integrity. The calorie-restriction theory of aging also has a tie to resveratrol.

Calorie restriction is currently the only proven method for extending life. It has been tested in as many as twenty-three species, including yeast, worms, flies, mice, and monkeys. Restricting calories means consuming about one-third fewer calories than would otherwise be consumed in the typical diet. Our species has evolved to suspend aging during times of scarcity, and calorie restriction works by tricking the body into thinking there is a famine.

Even though calorie restriction is based on a varied and nutritious diet, it remains a radical diet for humans. Realistically, few can sustain it, although members of groups like the Calorie Restriction Society are devoted to this practice, which can protect against heart disease, high blood pressure, high cholesterol, and type 2 diabetes.

But what if you could get all the benefits of calorie restriction without cutting calories? The good news is that resveratrol counteracts aging the same way that calorie restriction does, only without the deprivation. Resveratrol and calorie restriction both

People Are Living Longer

According to the Centers for Disease Control, the average American's life expectancy is now 77.9 years. One hundred years ago, the average typical life span was fewer than fifty years. One thousand years ago, it was fewer than twenty-five years. And life expectancy will continue to increase. Major breakthroughs, like a cure for cancer, may even accelerate the pace. But is there a limit to how old we can get? Evolutionary biologists estimate 120 years to be the maximum human life span. However, other scientists assert there may be no fixed limit to the number of years we can stay alive. Despite this scientific debate, it seems logical that if we make optimal lifestyle choices, we can extend our life expectancies within predetermined biological limits.

activate sirtuins, enzymes that regulate the body's defenses against aging and disease.

Longevity Genes and Sirtuin Enzymes

L ongevity genes are involved in the aging process. When they are stimulated by resveratrol or caloric restriction, positive effects on both aging and health result. Massachusetts Institute of Technology (MIT) researcher Lenny Guarente and his colleagues first discovered the longevity gene, called SIR2, which controls the aging process, in yeast. Similar genes are found in all living organisms. Humans have seven SIR2-like genes, which are referred to as SIRT1–7. The SIRT1 gene in mice is almost identical to the human version, so mice are often used as the subjects of longevity research. In addition to their work on yeast genes, Guarente's lab did research on calorie restriction and its effects on yeast and roundworms. They found that calorie restriction extended life spans in these lower organisms.

What do these discoveries in yeast, roundworms, and mice have to do with extending human life? In his book about this research, *Ageless Quest*, Guarente explains, "In the case of SIR2, there is a strong evolutionary case to be made that the gene may regulate survival in humans. The logic goes like this: Yeast and worms are very divergent evolutionarily, having separated from some common ancestor about one billion years ago, yet both use SIR2 to regulate survival. Any gene whose function has been conserved over that expanse of evolutionary time is very likely to have retained that role during the evolution of mammals, including humans. Evolution does not usually throw away something that serves a useful purpose."

As part of their natural function, cells turn on or turn off different genes. In Guarente's lab, researchers found that enzymes called sirtuins guard genes that should be turned off and ensure that they remain off. When the wrong genes are switched on, the cell can be damaged. Sirtuins also repair broken strands of DNA in the chromosomes. DNA, simply defined, is your unique genetic blueprint. When sirtuins leave their guard stations to repair DNA, genes are not regulated effectively, and cell performance declines. Over time, DNA damage can limit the cell's ability to regulate which genes are turned on and which are turned off. As a result, characteristics of aging set in.

David Sinclair, now a professor of pathology at Harvard Medical School, came from Australia to the United States to work as a postdoctoral fellow in Guarente's MIT lab during the 1990s, when the lab was at the forefront of longevity research. In 1999, Sinclair started his own laboratory at Harvard to study sirtuins. His work has been supported by the National Institute on Aging and other collaborators.

In 2003, Sinclair's lab identified several molecules that extend the life span of yeast cells. One of these turned out to be resveratrol, a substance that was already associated with the French paradox. Emerging as the most potent molecule in the study, resveratrol helped yeast cells live as much as 80 percent longer. This research made Sinclair the first to concretely link resveratrol and longevity.

The following year, Sinclair and his colleagues demonstrated that resveratrol slows aging in roundworms and fruit flies. Scientists in Italy later showed that large doses of resveratrol extend a typically short-lived fish's life span by up to 59 percent, depending on the dosage of resveratrol.

In a much-heralded 2006 study, Sinclair and his colleagues proved that resveratrol extends the life span of obese lab mice by triggering the longevity gene. Moreover, the mice became supermice, with better physical endurance and healthier organs than untreated mice. Rafael de Cabo of the National Institute on Aging and one of the study's lead investigators said, "After six months, resveratrol essentially prevented most of the negative effects of the high-calorie diet in mice." Sinclair added, "The 'health span' benefits we saw in the obese mice treated with resveratrol, such as increased insulin sensitivity, decreased glucose levels, and healthier heart and liver tissues, are positive clinical indicators and may mean we can stave off human age-related diseases such as type 2 diabetes, heart disease, and cancer, but only time and more research will tell."

It's important to note the significance of resveratrol's effect on high-fat diets. Obese mice were used because obesity tends to accelerate age-related diseases. It also is important to note that in this study mice were fed a huge daily dose of resveratrol, the equivalent of 750 to 1,500 bottles of red wine for a 150-pound person (depending on the wine's resveratrol content).

A 2009 study by Sinclair and a colleague unexpectedly showed that middle-aged mice treated with resveratrol acquired few diseases associated with aging but did not live longer than mice that were not treated with resveratrol. However, mice that were treated with resveratrol had less heart disease, stronger bones, fewer cataracts, and better motor function.

During the last decade, Sinclair's research has been featured in newspapers, magazines, and television programs around the world, and he has achieved a certain level of celebrity as a result. Frequently, media coverage focused on potential antiaging drugs that might be the ultimate result of such promising research. Indeed, versions of drugs that function like resveratrol by activating sirtuins are in the works.

Resveratrol and New Drugs

In 2004, Sinclair and his colleagues established Sirtris Pharmaceuticals in Cambridge, Massachusetts. In 2008, pharmaceutical giant GlaxoSmithKline bought Sirtris for $720 million. According to its website, Sirtris's mission is to discover and develop drugs that have the potential to treat diseases associated with aging. Potential drugs are designed to mimic the results of calorie restriction, without requiring a change in eating habits. The drugs feature synthetic versions of resveratrol, sirtuin activators that are up to one thousand times more potent than resveratrol. Therefore, these synthetic versions can be given in much lower doses.

Companies like Sirtris develop drugs to prevent or treat specific diseases. According to the Food and Drug Administration's definition, drugs must target specific diseases. Because aging is not a disease and no drug for aging is likely to be approved, no purely "antiaging" drug is in the pipeline. However, drugs designed to treat certain diseases may also have an antiaging effect.

In an early clinical trial involving people with type 2 diabetes, Sirtris's resveratrol formulation was shown to lower blood sugar and insulin. Another trial involving multiple myeloma was discontinued in May 2010 when some participants developed symptoms common to that ailment. This garnered negative press, even though most candidate drugs fail in clinical trials. Around the same time, even more controversy arose for Sirtris when another big pharma company reported that they could not replicate Sinclair's finding that resveratrol activates longevity genes.

Indeed, with so many disparate theories, aging research is a field that has seen much controversy over the years. Yet work being done in laboratories like Sirtris demonstrates that we are edging ever closer to finding the Fountain of Youth in pill form. We are no longer asking *if* we'll see such a breakthrough. Now we're asking *when*.

Nurture Trumps Nature

Ultimately, our best hopes for health and longevity may not be found in a laboratory. A flood of studies have shown that how we live our lives—what we believe, eat, do, and think—largely determines our health and longevity. In fact, our behaviors, lifestyles, and perspectives determine a whopping 70 percent of our longevity potential. Our genetic programming represents only 30 percent. So don't dismiss your chance of living well into old age if you happen to descend from an undesirable gene pool.

When we think about our lifestyle choices and how they will affect us over time, we acknowledge the obvious: We know we increase our odds of staying healthy and living long when we exercise consistently, get sufficient rest, and eat healthfully—and maybe even sip a little red wine. We recognize the wisdom of reducing stress, not smoking, and not drinking to excess. And we take common-sense precautions, like wearing seatbelts and getting preventive medical exams on schedule. Similar recommendations are repeated time and again in dozens of books about longevity that are now on the market. Of these books, those that give specific supplement recommendations include resveratrol on the list.

In one book, the author makes an observation about exercise that crystallizes its importance in a way that others have not. In *Younger Next Year for Women*, physician and coauthor Henry Lodge writes that aging is unstoppable, but decay is optional. From a biological prospective, *we either grow or decay*. To live long and well, we must send signals to our bodies and brains that we are in a growth phase. Regular exercise (six days a week) sends those signals. Some researchers think that exercise, like resveratrol and calorie restriction, activates longevity genes.

Less obvious contributors to health and longevity are the psychosocial aspects of life. A sense of connection and community—of belonging—is critical. People who age successfully live rich social lives and are active with family and friends. They work at creating and maintaining social networks. And they have positive attitudes and strong spiritual beliefs.

For humans, social interaction is essential. Dean Ornish, physician and founder of the Preventive Medicine Research Institute, emphasizes its importance in his book *Love and Survival*: "Anything that promotes a sense of isolation often leads to illness and suffering. Anything that promotes a sense of love and intimacy, connection and community, is healing."

On average, people include eight to eleven members in their personal networks. For people whose relationships are few and weak, the risk of death is two to four times as great, independent of all other factors (physical health, gender, race, socioeconomic status, and so forth).

Connectedness extends beyond human contact. Those who age successfully also report the benefits of interacting with nonhuman life forms, whether they be lovingly tended garden plants or beloved animal companions.

These words may best summarize this phenomenon: "If your heart doesn't have a reason to keep beating, it won't." This is a thought that Mehmet Oz, medical director, Integrative Medicine Program, NewYork-Presbyterian Hospital/Columbia University Medical Center and host of *The Dr. Oz Show*, occasionally shares with his audience.

Who Lives the Longest?

Blue Zones, a project funded by National Geographic and the National Institute on Aging, studies the world's longest-lived populations to identify lifestyle characteristics that can help people live longer, better lives. Researchers have identified the following Blue Zones, which

How to Live 122 Years

Jeanne Calment of Arles, France, died in 1997 at 122 years of age. She attributed her long life to drinking port wine, eating a lot of chocolate and olive oil, and bicycling and walking.

are geographic pockets where people consistently live the longest: Ikarìa, Greece; Loma Linda, California (home to Seventh-day Adventists); the Nicoya Peninsula, Costa Rica; Okinawa, Japan; and Sardinia, Italy.

Sardinians traditionally drink a red wine made from their native cannonau grapes, which develop a deep red pigment in response to the harsh Sardinian sun. Locals make their own wine and allow it to ferment with the skins for a long time. As a result, the wine is thought to have two to three times more flavonoids, such as resveratrol, than other wines.

Blue Zone researchers believe the following nine behaviors can promote longevity and greater quality of life:

1. Staying physically active, with consistent, moderate activity
2. Not eating until you feel full but stopping when you no longer feel hungry
3. Eating plant-based foods and avoiding meats and processed foods
4. Drinking red wine
5. Knowing your purpose in life
6. Taking time to relieve stress by slowing down, working less, resting
7. Participating in a spiritual community and having a feeling of belonging
8. Making family a priority
9. Creating a healthy social network by surrounding yourself with others who share Blue Zone values

The Older You Get, the Healthier You've Been

Researchers in the New England Centenarian Study use this phrase to contradict the myth that "the older you get, the sicker you get." In the United States, there are about 80,000 centenarians and sixty to seventy supercentenarians (age 110 and older). The U.S. Census Bureau has predicted that by the year 2050, there will be more than 800,000 centenarians in America.

Many centenarians remain free of disabilities until shortly before dying. About 90 percent remain physically and mentally healthy into their nineties. In fact, about 15 percent escape chronic illness altogether. Such exceptional health and longevity run very strongly in families.

In their book *Transcend*, authors Ray Kurzweil and Terry Grossman present the concept that if we live long enough, future technologies can extend our life spans even further. Bionic replacements, cloned organs, gene therapy, and nanotechnology may shape the medicine of tomorrow. As we await this remarkable marriage of biology and technology, we can design healthful lifestyles that will help us defy illness and aging. And resveratrol may be one bridge that helps us reach this new world of medicine.

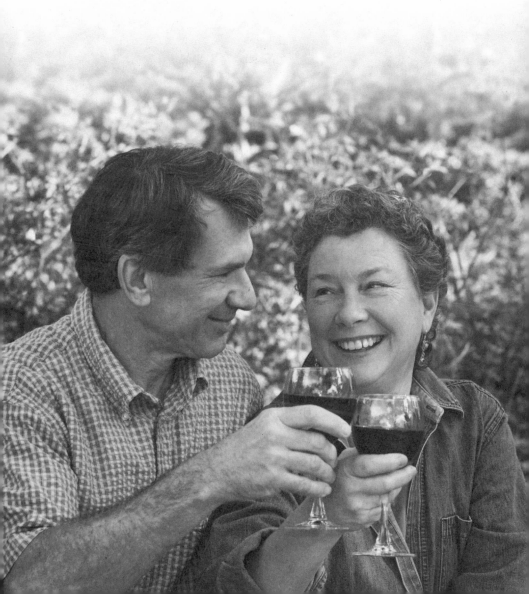

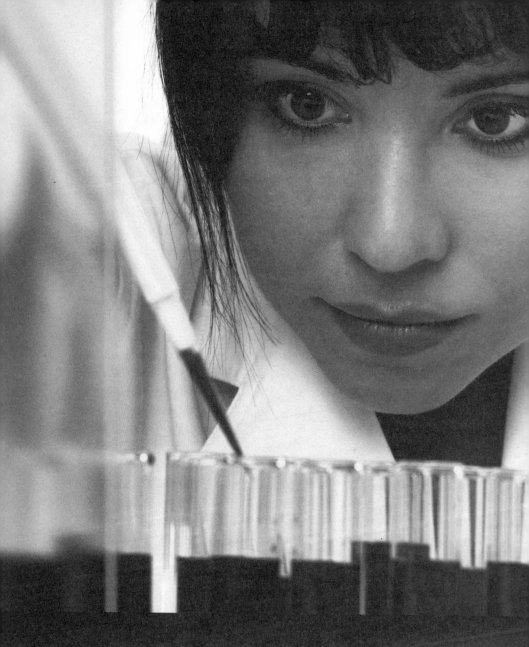

We need men who can dream of things that never were, and ask why not.

John F. Kennedy, 35th U.S. president, with a nod to George Bernard Shaw

Resveratrol and Medical Research

Resveratrol has been the subject of intense scientific interest in the past decade. The number of published, peer-reviewed studies involving resveratrol has skyrocketed from fewer than five hundred in the year 2000 to nearly thirty-five hundred today. These articles can be found in the U.S. National Institutes of Health online archive of biomedical and life sciences journal literature. With so much existing research on resveratrol, and with new information being published seemingly every day, there needed to be limits to what could be said in this book. Therefore, what follows is only a sampling to give you an idea of resveratrol's promise in preventing and treating disease.

Just as scientists have stood on the shoulders of their predecessors, this book relies on the work of researchers and journalists who have brought us the following information about resveratrol. This information is by no means complete and is not intended to replace the advice of your doctor.

Research regarding red wine's role in protecting us from cardiovascular disease appeared around 1992. By 1997, studies showing resveratrol's cancer-preventive properties dramatically increased interest in its potential. Today, heart disease, cancer, and stroke remain the three leading causes of death in the United States. Experts predict that sometime in the near future, cancer will overtake heart disease as the leading cause. Understandably, scientists are scrambling to find answers to the many questions surrounding these chronic and fatal conditions.

Resveratrol is a substance known to fight some of the worse attacks on our health. It is an antioxidant, as discussed in chapter 1. It also is known for its anti-inflammatory effects, which have considerable importance in reducing disease in our hearts, arteries, and brains. Resveratrol is also an effective antibacterial and antiviral agent, protecting us against contagion. And although aging is not a disease, resveratrol promises help in this area as well, with its potential to affect certain genes related to aging. Slowing down the aging process in turn can help us avoid the many chronic diseases associated with age.

In 2009, Lindsay Brown and his colleagues published a review of the resveratrol literature in the journal *Alcoholism: Clinical and Experimental Research*. The authors summarized what recent studies had to say about how resveratrol works and its potential therapeutic uses. Brown said the following about resveratrol: "The breadth of benefits is remarkable—cancer prevention, protection of the heart and brain from damage, reducing age-related diseases such as inflammation, reversing diabetes, and many more. It has long been a question as to how such a simple compound could have these effects, but now the puzzle is becoming clearer with the discovery of the pathways, especially sirtuins, a family of enzymes that regulate the production of cellular components by the nucleus."

Here are some of the highlights of the review:

- Resveratrol exhibits therapeutic potential for protecting us from cancer and heart disease.

- Resveratrol may aid in the prevention of age-related disorders, such as neurodegenerative diseases, inflammation, diabetes, and cardiovascular disease.

- Low doses of resveratrol improve *cell survival* in diseases of the circulatory and nervous systems, but high doses increase *cell death* when targeting cancer. It may seem contradictory that resveratrol can both protect and kill cells, but scientists attribute the different actions to dosage amounts.

Test Tubes and Animals

 uch of what science tells us about resveratrol is the result of *in vitro* studies, or research conducted in controlled environments. This kind of "test-tube" research often involves cell cultures. Considerable resveratrol research also is the result of *in vivo* studies, which involve live animals. Most clinical studies done on humans have been done on nonhuman animals first.

While research on animal models ultimately may help us discover how resveratrol can help humans, it's important to remember that results from animal studies should be considered cautiously. It's also very important to consider that animal studies often are performed with very high resveratrol doses. People could not get equivalent quantities by drinking red wine or even with heavy-handed supplement use. In fact, resveratrol research increasingly focuses on synthetic forms like those made by Sirtris Pharmaceuticals. These analogues have much higher potency than the natural form.

To date, we have limited results of human studies involving resveratrol. Over time, more research involving humans, including population studies, will provide the best understanding of resveratrol's potential. Stay tuned—important therapies may be just on the horizon.

Human Studies

The most prominent clinical trial involving resveratrol is for Sirtris Pharmaceuticals' proprietary formula, SRT501. This study of one hundred participants has shown that high doses of a synthetic form of resveratrol decreased blood sugar levels in people with diabetes. SRT501 was the first sirtuin activator proven to be safe and well tolerated in humans.

Joseph Maroon, physician and author of *The Longevity Factor*, and his colleagues conducted some of the first resveratrol research using human subjects. In a three-month study of fifty-one people, researchers found that a resveratrol supplement increased participants' endurance on a stationary bicycle. In addition, the supplement increased verbal memory scores on a standardized test.

In a June 2010 edition of the *American Journal of Clinical Nutrition*, researchers from Northumbria University described a clinical trial in which twenty-two adults were given resveratrol (a dose of either 250 or 500 milligrams) or a placebo on separate days. Forty-five minutes after taking the pill, participants were given a series of mental tasks. Those who had been given resveratrol had increased blood flow to the brain. When the larger dose of resveratrol was given, blood flow was greatest.

In mid-2010, the National Institutes of Health website, Clinical-Trials.gov, listed sixteen human studies involving resveratrol. These trials are in various stages, from recruiting to completion (for these, results have not yet been reported). The trials involve conditions such as Alzheimer's disease, cancer, and diabetes.

Cancer

In the United States, men have a one in two chance of developing cancer during their lifetimes. Women have a one in three chance. In cancer research, resveratrol is part of an important trend. About 70 percent of new chemotherapeutic agents are derived from natural products or synthetic versions based on their structures. Some researchers believe that resveratrol may be the most powerful naturally occurring anticancer substance known.

The earliest cancer research involving resveratrol focused on skin cancer. In the January 10, 1997, edition of the journal *Science*, researchers at the University of Illinois published a seminal paper reporting that when resveratrol is applied directly to the skin, it reduced the number of skin tumors in mice by up to 98 percent. In addition, the scientists were the first to describe the many ways that resveratrol can help prevent cancer. In research on the mice and on cancer cells, they found that resveratrol is effective in all three stages of cancer development: initiation, promotion, and progression. They also identified resveratrol as an antioxidant and an anti-inflammatory and found that it prevents the formation of new blood vessels that contribute to tumor growth.

Resveratrol inhibits cancer either by preventing enzymes from turning compounds into carcinogens or by regulating normal cell cycles. Following DNA damage, resveratrol can arrest cell activity to give the cell time to heal itself. If the damage cannot be repaired, resveratrol can stimulate the body's natural ability to destroy cancer cells. Notably, resveratrol induces cell death in a number of cancer cell lines (cancerous cells used in laboratory research). Resveratrol also inhibits the abnormal growth of cancer cells. Unlike normal cells, cancer cells grow rapidly and lose their ability to stimulate the body's defenses.

In a review published in the journal *Cancer Prevention Research* in May 2009, researcher Anupam Bishayee from the Northeastern Ohio

Resveratrol and Cancer

Resveratrol has been found to inhibit these cancers in human cell models and animals:

bone	liver	ovary
breast	lung	pancreas
cervical	lymphoma	prostate
colon	melanoma	squamous cell
esophagus	neuroblastoma	stomach
leukemia	oral cavity	thyroid

Source: *The Longevity Factor* by Joseph Maroon.

Colleges of Medicine and Pharmacy, offered this summary: "It is clear that resveratrol holds great potential not only in the prevention but also in the therapy of a wide variety of cancers. Tumor cells use multiple survival pathways to prevail over normal cells. . . . It may be speculated that resveratrol's anticancer effects cannot be explained by a unique mechanism of action but likely stem from various complementary actions." In addition, research studies have shown that resveratrol is an effective adjunct in various types of chemotherapy for different forms of cancer.

Breast Cancer

In 2008, University of Nebraska researchers reported that in test-tube studies resveratrol prevented estrogen from causing breast cancer. The formation of breast cancer is a multistep process that differs depending on various factors, including the type of disease and the patient's genetic makeup. However, scientists know that many breast cancers are fueled by increased estrogen.

"Resveratrol has the ability to prevent the first step that occurs when estrogen starts the process that leads to cancer. . . . We believe that this could stop the whole progression that leads to breast cancer down the road," said researcher Eleanor Rogan. She added that this discovery is particularly significant because fairly low concentrations of resveratrol were effective.

In the October 10, 2008, edition of the journal *Molecular Cell*, researchers discussed resveratrol's ability to reduce some inherited breast cancers caused by mutations in genes that suppress tumors.

They showed that resveratrol strongly inhibited this kind of tumor growth both in cultured cells and animal models.

Additional research has shown that resveratrol limits cell growth and promotes cell death on a highly invasive and metastatic cell line from human breast cancer. This type of breast cancer is resistant to several anticancer drugs.

Resveratrol was also found to be effective in animal studies that modeled breast cancer. Rats who were fed resveratrol throughout their lifetimes were less susceptible to mammary cancer. Resveratrol supplementation also reduced metastasis (spreading) of mammary tumors in rats.

Colon Cancer

Joseph Anderson and his colleagues at the University of New York at Stony Brook studied the development of colon cancer in 2,291 patients, comparing those who drank red wine and those who did not. The results showed that moderate wine drinkers were 45 percent less likely to develop colon cancer. Later research on the subject showed a 12 percent lower risk for white-wine drinkers and a 68 percent lower risk for red-wine drinkers. Researchers cite the high content of resveratrol in red wine as playing a key role.

In 2010, research out of the University of South Carolina's College of Pharmacy showed that resveratrol, when used in combination with other chemotherapy agents to treat colon cancer in mice, reduced tumor incidence from 80 percent to 20 percent. Researchers described resveratrol as a useful, nontoxic complementary and alternative strategy to reduce colon cancer.

Liver Cancer

Anupam Bishayee has noted that resveratrol has been well studied and shown to be effective for treating—but not preventing—liver cancer in animals. He and his colleagues are the first to demonstrate the preventive effects of resveratrol in relation to liver cancer. Dietary resveratrol inhibits the occurrence of liver cancer in rats.

Lung Cancer

Moderate consumption of red wine may decrease the risk of lung cancer in men, according to self-reported data from 84,170 men that was collected through the California Men's Health Study. Researchers measured the effect of beer, red wine, white wine, and hard liquor consumption on the risk of lung cancer. In 2008, they reported that red wine was most effective in reducing lung cancer risk and concluded that the antioxidant component in red wine may be the protective factor.

Pancreatic Cancer

In 2008, researchers from the University of Rochester Medical Center showed for the first time that resveratrol can help destroy pancreatic cancer cells. The study also showed that when pancreatic cancer cells were pretreated with resveratrol and then irradiated, the combination induced cell death, an important goal in cancer therapy.

Some physicians have expressed concern that antioxidants might end up protecting tumors, but this study showed there is little evidence to support that fear. Researchers said that, in this study, resveratrol seemed to make tumor cells more sensitive to radiation and make normal tissue less sensitive. In fact, in this research resveratrol not only reached its intended target by injuring the malignant cells but it also simultaneously protected normal tissue from the harmful effects of radiation.

Prostate Cancer

Researchers at the University of Alabama at Birmingham have found that resveratrol may help reduce the risk of developing prostate cancer. The study involved male mice who were given resveratrol with their food for seven months. These mice showed an 87 percent reduction in their risk of developing the most deadly kind of prostate tumor. Other mice in the study were also treated with resveratrol and developed a less-serious form of prostate cancer. However, compared to mice who were not treated with resveratrol, this group was 48 percent more likely to have their tumor growth halted or slowed. Other studies in which mice were given resveratrol through their drinking water showed that it suppressed prostate cancer growth and induced cell death.

Research results published in the *International Journal of Cancer* show that drinking a glass of red wine a day may cut a man's risk of prostate cancer in half and that the protective effect appeared to be strongest against the most aggressive forms of prostate cancer. Men who consumed four or more glasses of red wine per week have a 60 percent lower incidence of the more aggressive types of prostate cancer.

Other Cancers

Neuroblastoma is an aggressive childhood cancer that affects the nervous system and is very difficult to cure. In a 2004 issue of the magazine *Surgery*, researchers reported that they exposed neuroblastoma cells for varying lengths of time to a range of concentrations of resveratrol. The treatments resulted in a 70 percent increase in long-term cell survival, showing resveratrol to be a promising therapy.

Researchers at the University of Wisconsin School of Medicine say that resveratrol is a particularly promising treatment for young children because it's not toxic to healthy cells. Very young patients may live for a long time after their diagnosis, so potential treatments shouldn't cause other health problems. These researchers also have shown that resveratrol shrinks tumors and kills malignant cells in four other forms of cancer in mice: breast cancer, skin melanoma, and two cancers of the eye.

Diseases of the Circulatory System

Chapter 2 introduces the fact that modest consumption of red wine reduces risk of and death from cardiovascular disease, which includes disease of the arteries and blood vessels, heart disease, heart attack, and stroke. In the United States, cardiovascular disease accounts for one of every three deaths. Risk factors for cardiovascular disease include high blood pressure, obesity, and diabetes, as well as behaviors such as smoking or physical inactivity.

This chapter features research that shows how resveratrol protects the heart and the rest of the cardiovascular system. In a host of research studies, resveratrol has been shown to positively affect cholesterol levels, prevent damage to blood vessels (arteries and veins), reduce inflammation, and prevent and reduce blood clots by making it more difficult for platelets to stick together, thereby reducing heart attack risk. Early stages of cardiovascular disease include damage from free radicals, and because resveratrol is an antioxidant, it also contributes to cardiovascular health.

Resveratrol is helpful in maintaining healthful cholesterol levels. In 2005, researchers reported the results of a clinical study in *The Journal of Nutrition*. Participants included twenty-four premenopausal women and twenty postmenopausal women. All of the women were given a grape powder rich in resveratrol and other polyphenols for four weeks. At the conclusion of the study, all were found to have reduced levels of LDL ("bad") cholesterol and triglycerides. Other studies have shown that resveratrol can increase levels of HDL ("good") cholesterol. However, high cholesterol is but one part of the big picture in cardiovascular disease.

Healthy Blood Vessels

Healthy blood vessels (veins and arteries) are essential for cardiovascular health. As cardiovascular disease progresses, blood vessels may lose their ability to widen and contract (dilate), and blood may clot. An important player in this process is the endothelium, a specialized layer of cells that lines the interior surface of the blood vessels of the entire circulatory system, from the heart to the smallest capillary. The endothelium serves as the interface between circulating blood and the rest of the blood vessel. It controls blood pressure, blood clotting, and the formation of new blood vessels, as well as atherosclerosis, inflammation, and swelling. Although you may never have heard of the endothelium, if it does not function properly, cardiovascular disease will be the result. Resveratrol nourishes and helps to maintain the endothelium, supporting blood flow.

In the April 14, 2010, edition of the *American Journal of Clinical Nutrition*, researchers from Israel reported the results of a clinical study in which young, healthy participants drank a portion of red wine daily. Daily red-wine consumption for twenty-one days significantly enhanced vascular endothelial function.

Researchers have homed in on nitric oxide as a critical component in endothelial function. Nitric oxide allows blood vessels to relax. In animal studies, resveratrol has been shown to increase nitric oxide levels. And in a 2002 study published by The American Heart Association, human umbilical endothelial cells were treated with a red-wine extract, which led to an increase in nitric oxide levels. Researchers concluded that increased nitric oxide levels disrupt the development of endothelium dysfunction and atherosclerosis.

Atherosclerosis, Heart Attack, and Stroke

An encouraging study has shown that resveratrol in combination with other supplements can reduce the risk of heart attack; risk of heart attack increases as arteries become clogged with plaque. If uncontrolled, plaque will build up and form an atheroma, a fatty degeneration of the inner layers of the arteries. An atheroma (think of atherosclerosis) is thought to be the main factor in causing heart attacks. Studies conducted in Japan and Africa found that both populations had the same degree of atheroma as people in the United States but had statistically fewer heart attacks. This research suggested that blood clots rather than atheroma are the major cause of heart attacks.

Blood clots form when platelets aggregate, or stick together. This can lead to blocked arteries, heart attack, and stroke. Several studies have shown that resveratrol limits platelet aggregation and blood clotting. One researcher reported that resveratrol in combination with quercetin, selenium, and vitamins C and E also reduces platelet aggregation, encouraging better blood flow through the arteries.

University of Connecticut researchers showed that resveratrol prevents heart attacks and limits heart attack damage in mice who have been pretreated with resveratrol. Similarly, in April 2010, researchers at Johns Hopkins reported that resveratrol may protect against stroke. Two hours after feeding mice a single modest dose of resveratrol, researchers abruptly cut off their blood supplies, inducing ischemic stroke. Animals that had been pretreated with resveratrol suffered significantly less brain damage compared to those who had not. Researchers said the study adds to evidence that resveratrol can potentially build brain resistance to stroke. Their ongoing research also suggests some therapeutic benefits to giving resveratrol to mice after a stroke to limit further neuronal damage.

The March 12, 2009, edition of the *New England Journal of Medicine* included an article titled "Reversing Atherosclerosis?" The author discussed a study that examined how "foam cells" loaded with cholesterol become trapped in the innermost layer of an artery, contributing to atherosclerosis. When exposed to resveratrol, these cells were "untrapped," or remobilized, reversing disease risk.

In the United Kingdom, a playful report in the magazine *Men's Health* underscored just how important it is for arteries to remain open and flexible. The article suggested that because resveratrol works to enhance blood flow, it may in turn improve erectile function. Move over, Viagra.

Fruits and Veggies Reduce Heart Disease Risk

In a 2001 edition of the *Annals of Internal Medicine*, authors described a population study of 84,251 women from the Nurses' Health Study and 42,148 men from the Health Professionals' Follow-Up Study. They found that eating fruits and vegetables reduced heart disease risk in both

Resveratrol Instead of Aspirin?

Many people regularly take aspirin to prevent heart attacks and other cardiovascular illness. In 2005, Austrian researchers reported the results of a study in which they compared resveratrol, aspirin, and the drug atorvastatin (sold under the brand name Lipitor). Resveratrol showed similar effectiveness as the others. Other researchers found that resveratrol inhibited platelet aggregation in high-risk cardiac patients who could not tolerate aspirin. Thus, resveratrol may be an effective alternative cardioprotective agent for people who are aspirin sensitive.

women and men. The greatest reduction in risk was seen in those who ate eight servings per day; as few as four servings per day were associated with a slight but insignificant reduction in risk. These findings were similar to the researchers' earlier findings related to diet and stroke risk. In that study, published in the October 6, 1999, edition of the *Journal of the American Medical Association*, researchers reported that for each one-serving increase in daily fruit or vegetable intake, stroke risk was reduced by 6 percent. Cruciferous vegetables, green leafy vegetables, and citrus fruits and juices had the greatest protective effect.

There's no doubt that what we choose to eat greatly influences our heart health. In February 2006, Italian researchers reported in the *American Journal of Clinical Nutrition* that there are nine common risk factors for heart attack in people of almost every geographic region and in every racial group worldwide. Of these nine risk factors, eight are influenced by diet.

Diabetes and Obesity

For our ancestors, food was much more difficult to come by, and starvation and famine were real threats. Understandably, our bodies evolved to hold on to every bit of fat we could consume. Now, when food is plentiful, this genetic programming no longer serves us well. Storing too much fat in our bodies leads to obesity and obesity-related diseases like type 2 diabetes. As research with obese mice by David Sinclair and others have shown us, resveratrol has the potential for preventing or treating obesity in humans.

In the United States, nearly 34 percent of adults and 17 percent of children are obese. In addition, 68 percent of adults and nearly one-third of children are considered overweight. About 8 percent of the population (nearly 24 million people) has diabetes. Of these, only about 18 million people have been diagnosed. That leaves approximately 6 million Americans who have diabetes but don't know it. Type 2 diabetes, which represents 90 to 95 percent of all diabetes, is primarily caused by lifestyle factors. Type 1 diabetes is more closely linked to genetics.

People with type 2 diabetes are said to be insulin resistant, meaning the body can't use the insulin that it produces or that the body is not producing enough insulin. A hormone produced in the pancreas, insulin controls blood sugar (glucose) levels. The body needs insulin to regulate energy. In numerous studies using animals, resveratrol has been shown to affect insulin secretion and blood insulin concentrations. Resveratrol lowers insulin levels in the blood, among other positive effects.

In a 2008 article published in the journal *Biomedicine and Pharmacotherapy*, researchers summarized how resveratrol, when taken orally, showed antidiabetic effects in rats. Researchers gave rats 5 milligrams of resveratrol per kilogram of body weight. After thirty days, the rats showed markedly improved blood sugar levels and other positive effects. In fact, researchers concluded that resveratrol's effectiveness was comparable with gliclazide, an oral diabetes drug. They concluded the following: "The present findings suggest that resveratrol may be considered as an effective therapeutic agent for the treatment of diabetes mellitus."

In 2009, researchers from the University of Texas Southwestern Medical Center injected resveratrol directly into rats' brains. They found that resveratrol lowered insulin levels in the lab animals, even when the animals ate a high-fat diet. This research demonstrates the importance of resveratrol's action in the brain, specifically that it activates sirtuins there. This understanding may lead to the development of drugs that selectively target sirtuins in the brain to treat diabetes and potentially other conditions.

When our bodies efficiently manage blood sugar levels, we experience lower risk of cancer, dementia, heart disease, and secondary diagnoses related to diabetes. For example, diabetic neuropathy affects the body's nervous system, resulting in a multitude of symptoms. Researchers who treated rats with resveratrol found that it protected against various causes of diabetic neuropathy due to its antioxidant and anti-inflammatory effects.

Diabetes and Alcohol

Researchers have examined the link between alcohol consumption and diabetes. In 2004, the *Annals of Internal Medicine* printed a review of the existing literature. The authors concluded that, as for many other conditions, moderate alcohol consumption is associated with a decreased risk of diabetes, but heavy alcohol consumption is associated with an increased risk. However, the authors did not specify whether wine offered more protection than other types of alcohol.

Diseases of the Brain and Nervous System

Alzheimer's disease, a form of dementia, is one of the most feared conditions associated with aging. People who have the disease experience problems with mental functions like reasoning, remembering, and processing perceptions. They also experience loss of speech, changes in personality, impaired judgment, and a gradual decline in memory. We're not talking about the kind of memory loss that many older people humorously refer to as "senior moments." It's normal to forget where you put your keys, but it's not normal to forget what keys are for. It's normal if you can't recall the name of an acquaintance when you unexpectedly run into him, but it's not normal to fail to recognize close friends and family members.

The most common form of dementia, Alzheimer's disease is fatal and there is no known cure. Alzheimer's disease is progressive. Over time, people with the condition become unable to perform simple everyday tasks like dressing themselves or eating. Eventually, the disease leads to the failure of other body systems, causing death. More than 35 million people worldwide and 5.5 million people in the United States have Alzheimer's disease. By 2050, experts estimate there may be up to 16 million cases in the United States.

Many studies have connected aging, and particularly brain aging, with the action of free radicals. The oxidative damage done by free radicals has been linked to Alzheimer's disease. Chapter 1 provided detailed information about free radicals and oxidative damage, and resveratrol's role as an antioxidant.

Alzheimer's disease is characterized by the buildup of amyloid-beta peptides, or plaque, and neurofibrillary tangles in areas of the brain that are important for memory and learning. The presence of both plaques and tangles is essential for the diagnosis of Alzheimer's disease, which historically has been confirmed only after death when the brain is autopsied. New dyes and scanning technologies are changing this, making it possible for researchers to observe plaque in the living brain. This ability will play a critical role not only in diagnosing the disease but also in developing new treatments.

In 2005, researchers at the Litwin-Zucker Research Center for the Study of Alzheimer's disease reported that resveratrol decreases the buildup of amyloid-beta peptides and plaque. Decreasing the buildup could potentially decrease the onset of Alzheimer's disease.

In the February 2009 edition of the journal *Neurochemistry International*, researchers reported that when mice were fed clinical doses of resveratrol for forty-five days, plaque formation was diminished between 48 and 90 percent. This range represents effects seen in different regions of the brain.

In the November 2009 edition of the journal *Neurotoxicology*, researchers reported that resveratrol may slow the formation of amyloid plaques by as much as 90 percent. Furthermore, resveratrol induced clumps of amyloid plaques to come apart, showing that it may have the potential to break down existing plaque.

In the May 28, 2010, edition of the *Journal of Biological Chemistry*, researchers reported that resveratrol was able to selectively target the toxic amyloid-beta peptides that form plaque. This discovery means we can pick out the clumps of peptides that are bad and leave alone those that are benign.

Laboratory and animal research also show that synthetic forms of resveratrol are promising in the treatment of Alzheimer's disease. Because scientists at the University of Maryland have been so impressed with the results of clinical studies involving resveratrol, they are obtaining analogues of resveratrol that are twenty times more potent than the original compound. They theorize that resveratrol analogues may also be effective in fighting other amyloid-related diseases, like Parkinson's disease and Huntington's disease.

Numerous studies have shown that treatment with resveratrol can markedly reduce brain damage caused by stroke, seizure, and epilepsy. In young rats, resveratrol injections following traumatic brain injury protected the brain and decreased neuron loss. In addition, treatment with resveratrol decreased anxiety and increased memory in animals subjected to blunt head trauma. Other research has shown that when blood flow to the brain is stopped but then restored, renewed circulation may result in inflammation and oxidation. Brain damage can lead to cell death and severe disability. Resveratrol appears to protect the brain against this type of damage in ways similar to how it repairs the cardiovascular system.

Alzheimer's Disease and Alcohol

In 2006, researchers at Mount Sinai School of Medicine reported that in studies of mice, cabernet sauvignon prevented the generation of amyloid-beta peptides and reduced the deterioration of memory. Based on this animal study, researchers concluded: "Moderate wine consumption, within the range recommended by the FDA dietary guidelines of one drink per day for women and two for men, may help reduce the relative risk for AD clinical dementia."

In fact, studies have shown that drinking a little alcohol may reduce the risk of dementia and cognitive diseases. For example, in the May 22, 2007, edition of the journal *Neurology*, Italian researchers reported that they studied about 1,500 people ages sixty-five to eighty-four for more than 3.5 years. They found that those with mild cognitive impairment who had one drink per day progressed to dementia at a slower rate than those who drank no alcohol.

Alzheimer's Disease and Prevention

Research on centenarians shows that Alzheimer's disease is not an inevitable part of aging. The disease is the result of both genetic and environmental factors. However, researchers disagree about whether lifestyle choices can affect our risk for Alzheimer's disease.

Population studies have shown that people who consume greater amounts of fruits and vegetables, as well as vitamin supplement users, have lower rates of Alzheimer's disease. In one study supported by the National Institutes on Aging, vegetable consumption was associated with a reduced risk of cognitive decline in women.

If you don't like to eat your vegetables, studies show that drinking vegetable and fruit juices is a good alternative. In the September 2006 edition of *The American Journal of Medicine*, Vanderbilt University researchers reported findings from a large population study. They found that people who drank three or more servings of fruit and vegetable juices per week had a 76 percent lower risk of developing Alzheimer's disease than those who drank juice less than once per week.

In an article in the January 2010 edition of the journal *Archives of Neurology*, researchers reported the results of a six-month clinical trial involving adults ages fifty-five to eighty-five who had been diagnosed with mild cognitive impairment and who had an increased risk for developing Alzheimer's disease. At the conclusion of the study, those who participated in a structured exercise program were able to concentrate better and perform more-complex tasks than the control group. In addition, Harvard University psychiatrist and researcher John Ratey says there is overwhelming evidence that exercise, including leisure activities like painting and gardening, can preserve cognitive function and helps to fight dementia.

Red wine's potential for reducing Alzheimer's risk is supported by several observations. In 1997, the first study linked mild to moderate red wine consumption with decreased risk for the disease. A study of people age sixty-five and older confirmed that red wine, but not other types of alcohol, was associated with a low risk of dementia, including Alzheimer's disease. A Canadian population study determined that red wine consumption offered the most protection from Alzheimer's disease, reducing the risk by up to 50 percent.

The good news is that there may be ways that we can resist cognitive decline. After all, our brains change as the result of our experiences, continuously forming new brain cells and connective tissue throughout our lifetimes.

Parkinson's Disease

Actor Michael J. Fox, who has Parkinson's disease, has created a foundation for Parkinson's disease research. The foundation is currently funding a study involving resveratrol. Researcher Benjamin Wolozin at Boston University School of Medicine has found that natural resveratrol as well as a synthetic version from Sirtris can protect roundworms against Parkinson's disease. Because roundworms have the same protein that causes Parkinson's in people, this finding may lead to innovative new drugs for Parkinson's and other neurodegenerative diseases.

Researchers from China reported in the December 2008 *European Journal of Pharmacology* that resveratrol was given orally to rats with Parkinson's disease, daily for ten weeks. Results demonstrated that resveratrol reduced inflammation and had a neuroprotective effect.

Researchers in Quebec studied both resveratrol and another poly-phenol found in red wine, quercetin, and their effects on Parkinson's. In the lab, they found that both compounds helped to prevent a neuro-toxin that has been associated with Parkinson's from killing brain cells.

Resveratrol and Other Health Concerns

Eye Disease

In the July 2010 edition of the *American Journal of Pathology*, Washing-ton University School of Medicine researchers reported that resveratrol stopped the formation of damaging blood vessels in the eyes of mice and eliminated abnormal vessels that already had begun to develop. In the eye, blood vessel growth is associated with macular degeneration and diabetic retinopathy, so resveratrol may one day play a role in preventing these diseases. In addition, in research on cells, resveratrol has shown promise in preventing tissue abnormalities associated with glaucoma.

Depression

In experiments conducted on mice, resveratrol produced a significant increase in serotonin and noradrenaline levels. Researchers concluded that resveratrol has an antidepressant-like effect and potential thera-peutic value for people with depression.

Liver Disease

In the June 14, 2010, edition of the journal *Liver International*, Ohio researchers reported that resveratrol has shown considerable promise as a preventive and therapeutic agent in liver diseases, such as alco-holic cirrhosis, cancer, drug-induced toxicity, and viral hepatitis. Ear-lier animal studies showed that resveratrol helped to break down fat and remove it from the liver, making it a promising agent for prevent-ing or treating human *alcoholic* fatty liver disease. In another study, resveratrol decreased *nonalcoholic* fatty liver disease in rats.

Lung Disease

In 2010, Australian researchers published a paper discussing resveratrol's potential therapy in respiratory diseases, such as asthma and chronic obstructive pulmonary disease (COPD), which results in progressive breathlessness. These diseases involve airway inflammation that is triggered by allergens, viruses, and cigarette smoke. Activation of airway inflammatory cells results in oxidative stress. Therefore, an antioxidant like resveratrol may be useful in managing inflammatory airway disease.

In 2007, University of Rochester researchers reported their discovery that the toxins in cigarette smoke wipe out a longevity gene that protects the lungs from destructive inflammation and diseases such as COPD. They have begun to use resveratrol to develop a treatment to target the gene and reverse lung damage, or at least enhance the way standard COPD therapies work. Such a treatment could be a boon to smokers who are too addicted to quit and to those who have quit but remain at risk for lung disease as they age.

Earlier studies have shown that COPD progresses more slowly in moderate red-wine drinkers versus abstainers or heavy drinkers. Anti-inflammatory polyphenols, like resveratrol in red wine, may account for the beneficial effects on pulmonary function and a decline in the rate of progression of COPD.

Radiation

In test-tube experiments in which human cells were exposed to gamma radiation, resveratrol produced protective measures. Some of the cells were pretreated with resveratrol and some were not. In the resveratrol-treated group, 30 percent of the cells survived, as opposed to 10 percent of the untreated group. This is a promising finding given the lack of drugs that protect against or counteract radiation exposure.

Viruses and Bacteria

Scientists at the Institute of Microbiology in Rome have researched resveratrol's ability to fight the influenza virus. In influenza cell cultures, resveratrol strongly inhibited the replication of the virus. In another study, herpes virus cell growth was arrested one hour after administration of resveratrol. Both of these studies suggest that resveratrol reduces the production of the protein needed to regulate viral proliferation.

As an antiviral, resveratrol is effective in treating genital herpes topically, say researchers from Northeastern Ohio Universities Colleges of Medicine and Pharmacy. Resveratrol is also being studied for potential HIV treatment that targets cellular activity rather than the virus itself. In addition, resveratrol's immune-boosting properties are being studied in a clinical trial involving people with HIV.

Resveratrol also has been found to inhibit the growth of *Helicobacter pylori*, a bacteria that causes peptic ulcers, gastritis, and gastric cancers. The study compared muscadine grape-skin extract with pure resveratrol and other grape extracts. The muscadine grape-skin extract had the highest antibacterial effect. Pure resveratrol also inhibited *H. pylori*.

Women's Health

In research involving human bone marrow–derived cell cultures, resveratrol was found to have potential in preventing postmenopausal osteoporosis. Other studies have found resveratrol to be a potential alternative to hormone replacement therapy. By mimicking estrogen, resveratrol may be helpful in warding off menopause's many uncomfortable symptoms, such as hot flashes and night sweats.

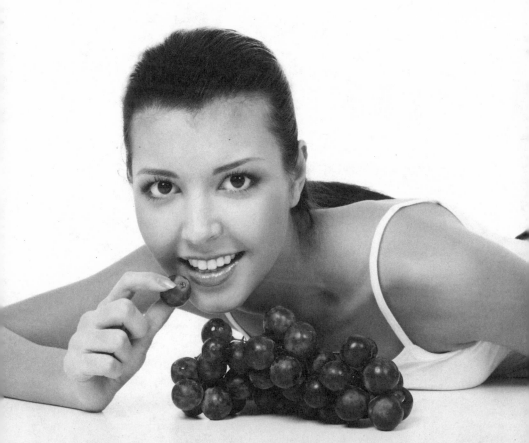

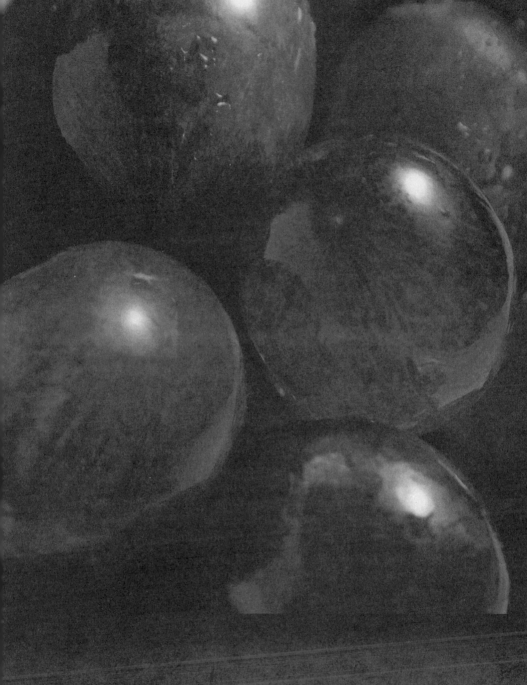

In Vino Veritas

Pliny the Elder, *Historia Naturalis*, 75 A. D.

Conclusion

I n 2003, David Sinclair linked resveratrol to longevity. In 2006, he and his colleagues showed that resveratrol extends the life span of lab mice by triggering the longevity gene. A media frenzy followed. Some cautioned that the furor was premature, yet our imaginations caught fire at the prospect of longer, healthier lives.

From ancient to modern times, the idea of immortality (or at least extremely long life), has perennially tantalized the human psyche. We need only look at popular tales—from the biblical Methuselah to the gods of Greek mythology, from the vampiric villains of folktales to comic-book superheroes—to find evidence of our innate and long-standing fascination with cheating death. The theme remains strong today in science fiction and fantasy, right down to the popular Harry Potter series in which the antagonist, Lord Voldemort, first sought the Philosopher's Stone and then employed forbidden horcruxes in a quest to become immortal.

There can be little wonder that our long-smoldering fascination would be flamed by the discovery of the miracle molecule resveratrol. Headlines in respected outlets, like *Fortune, Nature, Newsweek,* the *New York Times, Scientific American, Time,* and *U.S. News and World Report,* have reflected our fascination.

At the same time, the scientists featured in this extensive media coverage remind us that resveratrol research is in its infancy. We are only a few years in, albeit with thousands of peer-reviewed research articles attesting to resveratrol's very real promise. Clearly, the scientific community has responded swiftly and enthusiastically to resveratrol's potential and the wide range of positive effects it may have on our health and life span. It is worthy of their intense scrutiny, yet human studies have barely begun. There are still countless questions to pose about resveratrol. And there are still countless answers that can stimulate our interest even further.

While scientists do their thing, people who act as their own health advocates have their own steps to take. Certainly, resveratrol supplementation is one worth taking for folks on an antiaging program. Another important step is to stay abreast of health news. This task is aided and endlessly frustrated by the nature of our plugged-in society. We have access to much information—and misinformation—at our fingertips.

The good news is that the more inquisitive we are, the more we will see important themes emerge. For example, the long-lived cultures described briefly in this book share common behaviors. Many drink moderate amounts of wine. Most also enjoy a plant-based diet, get sufficient and sustained physical exercise, and are rewarded with a sense of belonging by engaging in their communities and with their families. By becoming students of longevity, by following the science and relying on reputable sources, we can develop our own workable formulations for extending our "health spans."

Maybe someday the fountain of youth and other tales of immortality will emerge from the pages of fiction. And perhaps someday soon, with the help of resveratrol, we really will live happily ever after—for a very long time.

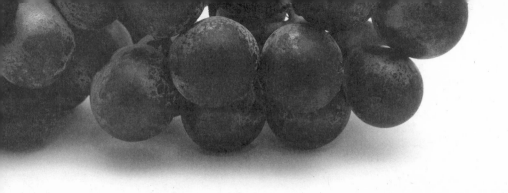

References

CHAPTER 1: Resveratrol and Antioxidants

Bliss, Rosalie Marion. 2007. "Nutrition and Brain Function: Food for the Aging Mind." *Agricultural Research*, August. www.ars.usda.gov/is/AR/archive /aug07/aging0807.pdf.

Bowden, Jonny. 2007. *The 150 Healthiest Foods on Earth*. Gloucester, MA: Fairwinds Press.

Carlsen, Monica, Bente Halvorsen, Kari Holte, et al. 2010. "The Total Antioxidant Content of More Than 3100 Foods, Beverages, Spices, Herbs, and Supplements Used Worldwide." *Nutr J* 9 (January 22):3.

Corti, Roberto, Andreas Flammer, Norman Hollenberg, and Thomas Luscher. 2009. "Cocoa and Cardiovascular Health." *Circulation* 119:1433–1441.

Gross, Paul. 2010. *Superfruits*. New York: McGraw-Hill.

Hollenberg, Norman, and Naomi Fisher. 2007. "Is It the Dark in Dark Chocolate?" *Circulation* 116:2360–2362.

Hollenberg, Norman, Naomi Fisher, and Marjorie McCullough. 2009. "Flavonols, the Kuna, Cocoa Consumption, and Nitric Oxide." *J Am Soc Hypertens* 3(2): 105–112.

Jeep, Robin, and Richard Couey. 2008. *The Super Antioxidant Diet and Nutrition Guide*. Charlottesville, VA: Hampton Roads Publishing.

Lee, K. W., Y. J. Kim, H. J. Lee, and C. Y. Lee. 2003. "Cocoa Has More Phenolic Phytochemicals and a Higher Antioxidant Capacity than Teas and Red Wine." *J Agric Food Chem* 51(25): 7292–7295.

Linus Pauling Institute, Oregon State University, Micronutrient Information Center. http://lpi.oregonstate.edu/infocenter/phytochemicals/resveratrol.

Manach, C., G. Williamson, C. Morand, A. Scalbert, and C. Remesy. 2005. "Bioavailability and Bioefficiency of Polyphenols in Humans. I. Review of 97 Bioavailability Studies." *Am J Clin Nutr* 81(Suppl): 230S–242S.

Maroon, Joseph. 2009. *The Longevity Factor: How Resveratrol and Red Wine Activate Genes for a Longer and Healthier Life*. New York: Simon and Schuster.

Parente, Matilde. 2009. *Resveratrol*. Salt Lake City, UT: Woodland Publishing.

Peanut Institute. 2000. "Peanuts Contain Significant Amount of Plant Compound That May Prevent Risk of Heart Disease and Cancer." News release, March 1. www .peanut-institute.org/news-and-information/downloads/20000301_resveratrol.pdf.

Presta, Michele Antoniuk. 2009. "Determination of Flavonoids and Resveratrol in Wine by Turbulent-Flow Chromatography-LC-MS." *Chromotographia* 69(Suppl 2): 167–173.

Scalbert, Augustin, Ian Johnson, and Mike Saltmarsh. 2005. "Polyphenols: Antioxidants and Beyond." *Am J Clin Nutr* 81(Suppl): 215S–217S.

U.S. Department of Agriculture. 2007. "Oxygen Radical Absorbance Capacity (ORAC) of Selected Foods." www.ars.usda.gov/sp2userfiles/place/12354500/data/orac/orac07.pdf.

Williamson, Gary, and Claudine Manach. 2005. "Bioavailability and Bioefficiency of Polyphenols in Humans. II. Review of 93 Intervention Studies." *Am J Clin Nutr* 81(Suppl): 243S–255S.

World Health Organization. 2008. "Fact Sheet 134: Traditional Medicine." www.who.int/mediacentre/factsheets/fs134/en/index.html.

Wu, Xianli, Gary Beecher, Joanne Holden, et al. 2004. "Lipophilic and Hydrophilic Antioxidant Capacities of Common Foods in the United States." *J Agric Food Chem* 52:4026–4037.

CHAPTER 2: Red Wine and Health

Abedin, Shahreen. 2009. "Seniors: Drink to Your Health." CNNHealth, Jan. 21. www.cnn.com/2009/HEALTH/01/21/seniors.alcohol.disability/index.html.

Allen, Naomi, Valerie Beral, Delphine Casabonne, et al. "Moderate Alcohol Intake and Cancer Incidence in Women." *J Natl Cancer Inst* 101(5): 296–305.

American Cancer Society. 2006. "Alcohol and Cancer." www.cancer.org/acs/groups/content/@healthpromotions/documents/document/acsq-017622.pdf.

———. 2009. "Even Moderate Alcohol Use Increases Risk of Certain Cancers in Women." www.cancer.org/docroot/NWS/content/NWS_1_1x_Even_Moderate_Alcohol_Increases_Risk_of_Certain_Cancers_in_Women.asp?sitearea=NWS&viewmode=print&.

———. 2010. "Alcohol Use and Cancer." www.cancer.org/Cancer/CancerCauses/DietandPhysicalActivity/alcohol-use-and-cancer?sitearea=PED.

American Heart Association. 2009. "Alcohol, Wine, and Cardiovascular Disease." www.americanheart.org/presenter.jhtml?identifier=4422.

BBC News. 2002. "World's 'Oldest Man' Dies." BBC News Online, Jan. 5. http://news.bbc.co.uk/2/hi/europe/1744097.stm.

Belleville, J. 2002. "The French Paradox: Possible Involvement of Ethanol in the Protective Effect Against Cardiovascular Diseases." *Nutrition* 18(2): 173–177.

Biello, David. 2006. "Forget Resveratrol, Tannins Key to Heart Health from Wine." *Scientific American*, Nov. 29.

Constant, J. 1997. "Alcohol, Ischemic Heart Disease, and the French Paradox." *Coron Artery Dis* 8(10): 645–649.

Corder, Roger. 2007. *The Red Wine Diet*. New York: Avery.

Curtiss, Linda. 2009. "Reversing Atherosclerosis?" *N Eng J Med* 360(11): 1144–1146.

Di Castelnuovo, Augusto et al. 2006. "Alcohol Dosing and Total Mortality in Men and Women." *Arch Intern Med* 166:2437–2445.

Ector, B. J., J. B. Magee, C. P. Hegwood, and M. J. Coign. 1996. "Resveratrol Concentration in Muscadine Berries, Juice, Pomace, Purees, Seeds, and Wines." *Am J Enol Vitic* 47(1): 57–62.

Feigelson, Heather. 2002. "Alcohol Consumption Increases the Risk of Fatal Breast Cancer." *JAMA* 286(17): 2143–2151.

Frankel, E. N, J. Kanner, J. B. German, E. Parks, and J. E. Kinsella. 1993. "Inhibition of Oxidation of Human Low-Density Lipoprotein by Phenolic Substances in Red Wine." *Lancet* 341(8852): 454–457.

Grønbæk, M., A. Deis, T. I. Sorensen, et al. 1995. "Mortality Associated with Moderate Intakes of Wine, Beer, or Spirits." *BMJ* 310:1165–1169.

Grønbæk, Morten, Ulrik Becker, Ditte Johansen, et al. 2000. "Type of Alcohol Consumed and Mortality from All Causes, Coronary Heart Disease, and Cancer." *Ann Intern Med* 133:411–419.

Johansen, Ditte, Karina Friis, Erik Skovenborg, and Morten Grønbæk. 2006. "Food Buying Habits of People Who Buy Wine or Beer: Cross Sectional Study." *BMJ* 332:519–522.

Karlamangla, Arun, Catherine Sarkisian, Deborah Kado, et al. 2008. "Light to Moderate Alcohol Consumption and Disability: Variable Benefits by Health Status." *Am J Epidemiol* 169(1): 96–104.

Kopp, Peter. 1998. "Resveratrol, a Phytoestrogen Found in Red Wine. A Possible Explanation for the Conundrum of the 'French Paradox'?" *Eur J Endocrinol* 138:619–620.

Kushi, L. H., E. B. Lenart, and W. C. Willet. 1995. "Health Implications of Mediterranean Diets in Light of Contemporary Knowledge. 1. Plant Foods and Dairy Products." *Am J Clin Nutr* 61(6 Suppl): 1407S–1415S.

———. 1995. "Health Implications of Mediterranean Diets in Light of Contemporary Knowledge. 2. Meat, Wine, Fats, and Oils." *Am J Clin Nutr* 61(6 Suppl): 1416S–1427S.

Latifi, Sadia. 2009. "Keen Cuisine: A Bar Snack That Protects Your Health?" *Psychology Today*, Jan. 1.

Lloyd-Jones, Donald, Robert Adams, Todd Brown, et al. 2010. "Heart Disease and Stroke Statistics 2010 Update: A Report from the American Heart Association." *Circulation* 121:e46–e215.

Maloof, Rich. n.d. "A Drink to Your Health." MSN Health. http://health.msn.com/health-topics/heart-and-cardiovascular/articlepage.aspx?cp-documentid=100159760&page=1.

Marano, Hara Estroff. 2004. "Drink to Your Health." *Psychology Today*, Oct. 22.

Miyagi, Y., K. Miwa, and H. Inoue. 1997. "Inhibition of Human Low-Density Lipoprotein Oxidation by Flavonoids in Red Wine and Grape Juice." *Am J Cardiol* 80(12): 1627–1631.

Mukamal, K. J., S. E. Chiuve, and E. B. Rimm. 2006. "Alcohol Consumption and Risk for Coronary Heart Disease in Men with Healthy Lifestyles." *Arch Int Med* 166:2145–2150.

Olivier, Rachel. 2008. "Red Wine Consumption and Associated Health Benefits, the Resveratrol Story." *Original Internist* 15(3): 119–126.

Opie, Lionel, and Sandrine Lecour. 2007. "The Red Wine Hypothesis: From Concepts to Protective Signalling Molecules." *Eur Heart J* 28:1683–1693.

Panagiota, N. Mitrou, Victor Kipnis, Anne Thiébaut, et al. 2007. "Mediterranean Dietary Pattern and Prediction of All-Cause Mortality in a U.S. Population: Results from the NIH-AARP Diet and Health Study." *Arch Intern Med* 167(22): 2461–2468.

Renaud, Serge. 1992. "Wine, Alcohol, Platelets, and the French Paradox for Coronary Heart Disease." *Lancet* 339(8808): 1523–1526.

Renaud, Serge, René Guéguen, Pascale Conard, et al. 2004. "Moderate Wine Drinkers Have Lower Hypertension-Related Mortality: A Prospective Cohort Study in French Men." *Am J Clin Nutr* 80(3): 621–625.

Siemann, E. H., and L. L. Creasy. 1992. "Concentration of the Phytoalexin Resveratrol in Wine." *Am J Enol Vitic* 43(1): 49–52.

Simopoulos, A. P. 2001. "The Mediterranean Diet: What Is So Special About the Diet of Greece? The Scientific Evidence." *J Nutr* 131(11 Suppl): 3065S–3073S.

Stein, Rob. 2009. "A Drink a Day Raises Women's Risk of Cancer, Study Indicates." *Washington Post*, Feb. 25.

Steinberger, Mike. 2009. "A Spoonful of Vino." *Slate*, March 5. www.slate.com /id/2211597.

Szmitko, Paul, and Subodh Verma. 2005. "Red Wine and Your Heart." *Ciculation* 111:e10–e11.

Thun, Michael, Richard Peto, Alan Lopez, et al. 1997. "Alcohol Consumption and Mortality Among Middle-Aged and Elderly U.S. Adults." *N Eng J Med* 337(24): 1705–1713.

Tims, Dana. 2010. "Visionary Drives Williamette Valley Vineyards." *Oregonian*, Feb. 19.

Trichopoulou, Antonia. 2009. "Anatomy of Health Effects of the Mediterranean Diet: Greek EPIC Prospective Cohort Study." *BMJ* 338:b2337.

Willett, W. C., F. Sacks, A. Trichopoulou, et al. 1995. "Mediterranean Diet Pyramid: A Cultural Model for Healthy Eating." *Am J Clin Nutr* 61(6 Suppl): 1402S–1406S.

Zern, Tosca, and Maria Luz Fernandez. 2005. "Cardioprotective Effects of Dietary Polyphenols." *J Nutr* 135:2291–2294.

Zern, Tosca, Richard Wood, Christine Green, et al. 2005. "Grape Polyphenols Exert a Cardioprotective Effect in Pre- and Postmenopausal Women by Lowering Plasma Lipids and Reducing Oxidative Stress." *J Nutr* 135:1911–1917.

CHAPTER 3: Resveratrol Supplements

ABC News. 2010. "Fake News Sites Used to Pitch Products." KGO-TV, San Francisco, Aug. 31. http://abclocal.go.com/kgo/story?section=news/7_on _your_side&id=6992473.

Arnquist, Sarah. 2009. "With Resveratrol, Buyer Beware." *New York Times*, Aug. 18.

Aubrey, Allison. 2009. "Red Wine Pills: Buyer Beware." NPR, March 27. www.npr .org/templates/story/story.php?storyId=16304978.

Cobiella, Kelly. 2009. "Buyer Beware: Web Supplement Scams." CBS Evening News, July 29. www.cbsnews.com/stories/2009/07/28/eveningnews/main5193515 .shtml?tag=mncol;lst;1.

ConsumerLab.com. 2010. "Resveratrol Supplements," Product review, May 17.

ConsumerLab.com. 2010. "Vitamin D and Resveratrol Use Surge." News release, Feb. 1. www.consumerlab.com/news/Supplement_Survey_Report/01_31_2010.

Federal Trade Commission. "Facts for Consumers: Test Your Supplement Savvy." www.ftc.gov/bcp/edu/pubs/consumer/health/hea09.shtm.

Harris, Gardiner. 2010. "Study finds Supplements Contain Contaminants." *New York Times*, May 25.

Hobson, Katherine. 2010. "Resveratrol and CoQ10 Supplements Are Popular But Unproven." *U.S. News and World Report*, Feb. 12.

Johannes, Laura. 2009. "Toast to Your Health with a Supplement." *Wall Street Journal*, Dec. 22.

Kurzweil, Ray, and Terry Grossman. 2004. *Fantastic Voyage: Live Long Enough to Live Forever*. Emmaus, PA: Rodale.

Linus Pauling Institute, Oregon State University, Micronutrient Information Center. http://lpi.oregonstate.edu/infocenter/phytochemicals/resveratrol.

Maroon, Joseph. 2009. *The Longevity Factor: How Resveratrol and Red Wine Activate Genes for a Longer and Healthier Life*. New York: Simon and Schuster.

Morago, Greg. 2010. "Juices Can Pave Way to a Buff Body." *Houston Chronicle*, Feb. 25.

Oprah.com. 2009. "The Truth About Oprah, Dr. Oz, Acai, Resveratrol, Colon Cleanse and More." New release, Aug. 19. www.oprah.com/health/The-Truth-About -Oprah-Dr-Oz-Acai-Resveratrol-and-Colon-Cleanse.

Schardt, David. 2009. "Web Self-Defense: How to Protect Yourself Against Internet Scams." *Nutrition Action Newsletter*, April.

Smillie, Dirk. 2009. "A Headache for Dr. Oz." *Forbes*. www.forbes.com/forbes/2009 /0713/marketing-oprah-resveratrol-headache-for-doctor-oz.html.

Wade, Nicholas. 2006. "Yes, Red Wine Holds Answer. Check Dosage." *New York Times*, Nov. 2.

Walters, Barbara. 2009. "Barbara Walters' Statement on Resveratrol." ABC News, June 19. http://abcnews.go.com/2020/story?id=7876211&page=1.

Washington State Office of the Attorney General. 2009. "Consumer Alert: Consumers Juiced by Deceptive Acai and Resveratrol Product Ads." News release, Aug. 28. www.atg.wa.gov/pressrelease.aspx?&id=23712.

Weil, Andrew. 2009. "Can't Drink Enough Red Wine?" drweil.com. www.drweil .com/drw/u/QAA400541/Cant-Drink-Enough-Red-Wine.html?print=1.

Weintraub, Arlene. 2009. "Resveratrol: The Hard Sell on Anti-Aging." *Business Week*, March 9.

CHAPTER 4: The New Fountain of Youth

Arnette, Robin. 2009. "Aging Research Yields Promising Medical Compounds." Environmental Factor, September. www.niehs.nih.gov/news/newsletter/2009/september /docs/efactor.pdf.

Baard, Mark. 2009. "Age-Old Woes, New Tactics." *Boston Globe*, Oct. 19.

Baur, Joseph. 2009. "Biochemical Effects of SIRT1 Activators." *Biochim Biophys Acta* 1804(8): 1626–1634.

———. 2010. "Resveratrol, Sirtuins, and the Promise of a DR Mimetic." *Mech Ageing Dev* 131(4): 261–269.

Baur, Joseph, Kevin Pearson, Nathan Price, et al. 2006. "Resveratrol Improves Health and Survival of Mice on a High-Calorie Diet." *Nature* 444(7117): 337–342.

Boston University School of Medicine. n.d. "Why Study Centenarians? An Overview." The New England Centenarian Study. www.bumc.bu.edu/centenarian/overview.

Buettner, Dan. 2008. *The Blue Zone: Lessons for Living Longer from the People Who've Lived the Longest*. Washington, DC: National Geographic Society.

Butler, Robert. 2010. *The Longevity Prescription: The 8 Proven Keys to a Long, Healthy Life*. New York: Avery.

Callahan, Maureen. 2010. "Mortal Combat." *New York Post*, Feb. 21.

Crowley, Chris, and Henry Lodge. 2005. *Younger Next Year for Women*. New York: Workman Publishing.

Das, D. K., S. Mukherjee, and D. Ray. 2010. "Resveratrol and Red Wine, Healthy Heart, and Longevity." *Heart Fail Rev* 15(5): 467–477.

Day, Jennifer Cheeseman. 1996. *Population Projections of the United States by Age, Sex, Race, and Hispanic Origin: 1995 to 2050.* U.S. Bureau of the Census, Current Population Reports, P25-1130. Washington, DC: U.S. Government Printing Office.

Duncan, David Ewing. 2008. "Is Wine What Flows through the Fountain of Youth?" *Discover*, October.

Fontana, Luigi, and Samuel Klein. 2007. "Aging, Adiposity, and Calorie Restriction." *JAMA* 297:986–994.

Fusco, D., G. Colloca, M. R. Lo Monaco, and M. Cesari. 2007. "Effects of Antioxidant Supplementation on the Aging Process." *Clin Interv Aging* 2(3): 377–387.

Guarente, Lenny. 2003. *Ageless Quest: One Scientist's Search for Genes That Prolong Youth.* New York: Cold Spring Harbor Laboratory Press.

Harvard Medical School. 2008. "Researchers Identify a Potentially Universal Mechanism of Aging." News release, Nov. 26. http://web.med.harvard.edu/sites/RELEASES/html/112608_sinclair.html.

Kelly, Jack. 2009. "Physician Authors Share What They Know About Red Wine, Fitness." *Pittsburgh Post-Gazette*, Jan. 14.

Kurzweil, Ray, and Terry Grossman. 2004. *Fantastic Voyage: Live Long Enough to Live Forever.* Emmaus, PA: Rodale.

———. 2009. *Transcend: Nine Steps to Living Well Forever.* New York: Rodale.

Lagouge, M., C. Argmann, Z. Gerhart-Hines, et al. 2006. "Resveratrol Improves Mitochondrial Function and Protects Against Metabolic Disease." *J Cell* 127:1109–1122.

Liponis, Mark. 2007. *Ultralongevity: The Seven-Step Program for a Younger, Healthier You.* New York: Little Brown and Company.

Lyon, Lindsay. 2009. "Scientists Are Changing the Definition of 'Old Age.'" *U.S. News and World Report*, Dec. 23.

Markus, M. Andrea, and Brian Morris. 2008. "Resveratrol in Prevention and Treatment of Common Clinical Conditions of Aging." *Clinical Interventions in Aging* 3(2): 331–339.

Minino, Arialdi, Jiaquan Xu, Kenneth Kochanek, and Betzaida Tejada-Vera. 2007. "Death in the United States." National Center for Health Statistics. www.cdc.gov/nchs/data/databriefs/db26.pdf.

National Institute on Aging. 2006. "Study Demonstrates Improved Health, Survival in Aged Overweight Male Mice on Resveratrol." News release, Nov. 1. www.nih.gov/news/pr/nov2006/nia-01.htm.

———. 2008. "Resveratrol Found to Improve Health, But Not Longevity in Aging Mice on Standard Diet." News release, July 3. www.nih.gov/news/health/jul2008/nia-03.htm.

Ornish, Dean. 1998. *Love and Survival: The Scientific Basis for the Healing Power of Intimacy.* New York: HarperCollins.

Pearson, Kevin, Joseph Baur, Kaitlyn Lewis, et al. 2008. "Resveratrol Delays Age-Related Deterioration and Mimics Transcriptional Aspects of Dietary Restriction Without Extending Lifespan." *Cell Metab* 8(2): 157–168.

Powell, Alvin. 2007. "Harvard Researchers Find Longevity, Restricted Diet Link." *HarvardScience*, Sept. 20. www.harvardscience.harvard.edu/medicine-health/articles/harvard-researchers-find-longevity-restricted-diet-link?view=print.

Rimas, Andrew. 2006. "His Research Targets the Aging Process." *Boston Globe*, Dec. 11.

Roizen, Michael, and Mehmet Oz. 2005. *You: The Owner's Manual.* New York: HarperCollins.

Rowe, John Wallis, and Robert Kahn. 1998. *Successful Aging.* New York: Dell Publishing.

Rush University Medical Center. 2010. "Tangney and Colleagues Find That Diet May Slow Cognitive Decline." News release, May 3. www.rushu.rush.edu.

Schmidt, Charlie. 2010. "GSK/Sirtris Compounds Dogged by Assay Artifacts." *Nature Biotechnol* 28(3): 185–186.

Sinclair, David, and Lenny Guarente. 2006. "Unlocking the Secrets of Longevity Genes." *Scientific American,* Feb. 20.

Sirtris Pharmaceuticals. 2008. "Sirtris Announces SRT501 Lowers Glucose in Twice-Daily Dosing Clinical Trial; Study Suggests Dose Response for Proprietary Formulation of Resveratrol in Type 2 Diabetes." News release, April 17. http://sirtrispharma.com/press/2008-041708.html.

Stipp, David. 2007. "Drink Wine and Live Longer." *Fortune,* Feb. 23.

Time.com. 2010. "Health Checkup: How to Live 100 Years." Special series by multiple authors. www.time.com/time/specials/packages/completelist/0,29569,1963392,00.html.

Underwood, Anne. 2008. "Never Say Die." *Newsweek,* Dec. 6.

Wade, Nicholas. 2006. Yes, Red Wine Holds Answer. Check Dosage. *New York Times,* Nov. 2.

———— 2008. "Scientists Find Clues to Aging in a Red Wine Ingredient's Role in Activating a Protein." *New York Times,* Nov. 27.

———— 2009. "Tests Begin on Drugs That May Slow Aging." *New York Times,* Aug. 18.

———— 2009. "Quest for a Long Life Gains Scientific Respect." *New York Times,* Sept. 29.

Walters, Barbara. 2008. "Live to 150, Can You Do It?" ABC News, April 1. http://abcnews.go.com/print?id=4544003.

Whitney, Craig. 1997. "Jeanne Calment, World's Elder, Dies at 122." *New York Times,* Aug. 5.

CHAPTER 5: Resveratrol and Medical Research

Advanced Cardiology Institute. 2010. "Cardiologists Comment on Aspirin Versus Resveratrol." News release, Feb. 26. www.prnewswire.com/news-releases /cardiologists-comment-on-aspirin-versus-resveratrol-85463852.html.

Ajmo, J. M., X. Liang, C. Q. Rogers, B. Pennock, and M. You. 2008. "Resveratrol Alleviates Alcoholic Fatty Liver in Mice." *Am J Physiol Gastrointest Liver Phsyiol* 295(4): G833–G842.

American Association for Cancer Research. 2008. "Red Wine May Lower Lung Cancer Risk." www.aacr.org/home/public--media/aacr-press-releases/press-releases-2008 .aspx?d=1140.

————. 2008. "Researchers Identify Cancer Preventive Properties in Common Dietary Supplement." www.aacr.org/home/public--media/aacr-press-releases /press-releases-2008.aspx?d=1101.

American Cancer Society. 2010. *Cancer Facts and Figures 2010.* Atlanta: American Cancer Society.

Anderson, J. et al. 2006. Lifestyle or Resveratrol? Comparison of White and Red Wine Consumption and Colorectal Neoplasia. Proceedings from the 2006 annual meeting of the American College of Gastroenterology in Las Vegas, NV. Abstract 920.

Athar, Mohammed, Jung Ho Back, Xiuwei Tang, et al. 2007. "Resveratrol: A Review of Preclinical Studies of Human Cancer Prevention." *Toxicol Appl Pharmacol* 224(3): 247–283.

Aziz, Moammir, Minakshi Nihal, Vivian Fu, David Jarrard, and Nihal Ahmad. 2006. "Resveratrol-Caused Apoptosis of Human Prostate Carcinoma LNCaP Cells Is Mediated via Modulation of Phosphatidylinositol 3-kinase/Akt Pathway and Bcl-2 Family Proteins." *Mol Cancer Ther* 5(5): 1335–1341.

Baker, Laura, Laura Frank, Karen Foster-Schubert, et al. 2010. "Effects of Aerobic Exercise on Mild Cognitive Impairment." *Arch Neurology* 67(1): 71–79.

Baur, Joseph, and David Sinclair. 2006. "Therapeutic Potential of Resveratrol: The In Vivo Evidence." *Nature Rev Drug Discovery* 5:493–506.

BBC News. 2000. "Red Wine Can Stop Herpes." BBC News Online, Sept. 19. http://news.bbc.co.uk/2/hi/health/931850.stm.

Belluck, Pam. 2010. "Obesity Rates Hit Plateau in U.S., Data Suggest." *New York Times*, Jan. 14.

Bernstein, Lenny. 2010. "A Growing Body of Evidence Links Exercise and Mental Acuity." *Washington Post*, May 25.

Bhat, Krishna, Daniel Lantvit, Konstantin Christov, et al. 2001. "Estrogenic and Antiestrogenic Properties of Resveratrol in Mammary Tumor Models." *Cancer Res* 51:7456–7463.

Bishayee, Anupam. 2009. "Cancer Prevention and Treatment with Resveratrol: From Rodent Studies to Clinical Trials." *Cancer Prev Res* 2(5): 409–418.

———. 2009. "Resveratrol-Mediated Chemoprevention of Diethylnitrosamine-Initiated Hepatocarcinogenesis: Inhibition of Cell Proliferation and Induction of Apoptosis." *Chem Biol Interact* 179(2–3): 131–144.

———. 2010. "Resveratrol and Liver Disease: From Bench to Bedside and Community." *Liver Int* 30(8): 1103–1114.

———. 2010. "Resveratrol in the Chemoprevention and Treatment of Hepatocellular Carcinoma." *Cancer Treat Rev* 36(1): 43–53.

Brown, L., P. A. Kroon, D. K. Das, et al. 2009. "The Biological Responses to Resveratrol and Other Polyphenols from Alcoholic Beverages." *Alcohol Clin Exp Res* 33(9): 1513–1523.

Bujanda, Luis, Elizabeth Hijona, Mikel Larzabal, et al. 2008. "Resveratrol Inhibits Nonalcoholic Fatty Liver Disease in Rats." *BMC Gastroenterol* 8:40.

ClinicalTrials.gov. List of clinical trials involving resveratrol. www.clinicaltrials.gov/ct2/results?term=resveratrol. Accessed March 31, 2010.

Cui, Xiangli, Yu Jin, Anne Hofseth, et al. 2010. "Resveratrol Suppresses Colitis and Colon Cancer Associated with Colitis." *Cancer Prev Res* 3(4): 549–559.

Curtiss, Linda. 2009. "Reversing Atherosclerosis?" *N Eng J Med* 360(11): 1144–1146.

Dai, Z. 2007. "Resveratrol Enhances Proliferation and Osteoblastic Differentiation in Human Mesenchymal Stem Cells via ER-Dependent ERK1/2 Activation." *Phytomedicine* 14(12): 806–814.

Davis, C. et al. 2000. The Synergistic Inhibition of HIV-1 with Nucleoside Analogs Combined with a Natural Product, Resveratrol. Paper presented at the 7th Conf Retrovir Oppor Infect, Jan. 30–Feb. 2, San Francisco, CA.

De Caterina, Raffaele, Antonella Zampolli, Serena Del Turco, Rosalinda Madonna, and Marika Massaro. 2006. "Nutritional Mechanisms That Influence Cardiovascular Disease." *Am J Clin Nutr* 83(2): 421S–426S.

Deng, Chu-Xia et al. 2008. "New Findings May Improve Treatment of Inherited Breast Cancer." *Cell Press*, Oct. 11.

Desai, A., G. Grossberg, and J. Chibnall. 2010. "Healthy Brain Aging: A Road Map." *Clin in Geriatr Med* 26(1): 1–16.

Edwards, Scott. 2010. "Neuroprotection: Guarding Against Injury and Degeneration." The DANA Foundation. www.dana.org/news/publications/detail.aspx?id=24572.

Elliot, P. J., and M. Jirousek. 2008. "Sirtuins: Novel Targets for Metabolic Disease." *Curr Opin Investig Drugs* 9(4): 371–378.

Feng, Y., X. P. Wang, S. G. Yang, et al. 2009. "Resveratrol Inhibits Beta-Amyloid Oligomeric Cytotoxicity But Does Not Prevent Oligomer Formation." *Neurotoxicology* 30(6): 986–995.

Filomeni, G., I. Graziani, G. Rotilio, and M. R. Ciriolo. 2007. "Trans-Resveratrol Induces Apoptosis in Human Breast Cancer Cells MCF-7 by Activation of MAP Kinases Pathway." *Genes Nutr* 2:295–305.

Frampton, Gabriel, Eric Lazcano, Huang Li, Akimuddin Mohamad, and Sharon De-Morrow. 2010. "Resveratrol Enhances the Sensitivity of Cholangiocarcinoma to Chemotherapeutic Agents." *Lab Invest* 90:1335–1338.

Gaffney, Jacob. 2009. "Recent Research Bolsters Red-Wine Compound's Health Potential." *Wine Spectator*, July 6. www.winespectator.com/webfeature/show /id/Recent-Research-Bolsters-Red-Wine-Compounds-Health-Potential_4906.

Gill, C., S. E. Walsh, C. Morrissey, J. M. Fitzpatrick, and R. W. Watson. 2007. "Resveratrol Sensitizes Androgen Independent Prostate Cancer Cells to Death-Receptor Mediated Apoptosis through Multiple Mechanisms." *Prostate* 67(15): 1641–1645.

Hamed, Saher, Jonia Alshiek, Anat Aharon, Benjamin Brenner, and Ariel Roguin. 2010. "Red Wine Consumption Improves In Vitro Migration of Endothelial Progenitor Cells in Young, Healthy Individuals." *Am J Clin Nutr* 92:161–169.

Howard, Andrea, Julia Arnsten, and Marc Gourevitch. 2004. "Effect of Alcohol Consumption on Diabetes Mellitus." *Ann Intern Med* 140:211–219.

Hsieh, T. C., and J. M. Wu. 1999. "Differential Effects on Growth, Cell Cycle Arrest, and Induction of Apoptosis by Resveratrol in Human Prostate Cancer Cell Lines." *Exp Cell Res* 249(1): 109–115.

Jang, M., G. O. Udeani, K. V. Slowing, et al. 1997. "Cancer Chemopreventive Activity of Resveratrol, a Natural Product Derived from Grapes." *Science* 275:218–220.

Johns Hopkins Medicine. 2010. "How Red Wine May Shield Brain from Stroke Damage." News release, April 21. www.hopkinsmedicine.org/Press_releases /2010/04_21a_10.html.

Joshipura, K. J., A. Ascherio, J. E. Manson, et al. 1999. "Fruit and Vegetable Intake in Relation to Risk of Ischemic Stroke." *JAMA* 282:1233–1239.

Kamholz, Stephan. 2006. "Wine, Spirits, and the Lung: Good, Bad, or Indifferent?" *Trans Am Clin Climatol Assoc* 117:129–145.

Kennedy, David, Emma Wightman, Jonathon Reay, et al. 2010. "Effects of Resveratrol on Cerebral Blood Flow Variables and Cognitive Performance in Humans: A Double-Blind, Placebo-Controlled, Crossover Investigation." *Am J Clin Nutr* 91:1590–1597.

Kolata, Gina. 2010. "Promise Seen for Detection of Alzheimer's." *New York Times*, June 23.

Lu, Fang, Muhammad Zahid, Cheng Wang, et al. 2008. "Resveratrol Prevents Estrogen-DNA Adduct Formation and Neoplastic Transformation in MDF-10F Cells." *Cancer Prev Res* 1 (July):135–145.

Luna, C., G. Li, P. B. Liton, et al. 2008. "Resveratrol Prevents the Expression of Glaucoma Markers Induced by Chronic Oxidative Stress in Trabecular Meshwork Cells." *Food Chem Toxicol* 47(1): 198–204.

Luther, D. J., V. Ohanyan, P. E. Shamhart, et al. 2009. "Chemopreventive Doses of Resveratrol Do Not Produce Cardiotoxicity in a Rodent Model of Hepatocellular Carcinoma." *Invest New Drugs*, Oct. 8 (Epub ahead of print).

Marambaud, Philippe, Haitian Zhao, and Peter Davies. 2005. "Resveratrol Promotes Clearance of Alzheimer's Disease Amyloid-Beta Peptides." *J Biol Chem* 280(45): 37377–37382.

Marino, Melissa. 2006. "Study Finds Juice May Help Reduce Alzheimer's Risk." *Reporter* (Vanderbilt University Medical Center Weekly Newspaper), Sept. 1.

Markus, M. Andrea, and Brian Morris. 2008. "Resveratrol in Prevention and Treatment of Common Clinical Conditions of Aging." *Clinical Interventions in Aging* 3(2): 331–339.

Maroon, Joseph. 2009. *The Longevity Factor: How Resveratrol and Red Wine Activate Genes for a Longer and Healthier Life*. New York: Simon and Schuster.

National Cancer Institute. "Red Wine and Cancer Prevention: Fact Sheet." www.cancer.gov/cancertopics/factsheet/prevention/redwine.

Pal, Sebely, Nerissa Ho, Carlos Santos, et al. 2003. "Red Wine Polyphenolics Increase LDL Receptor Expression and Activity and Suppress the Secretion of ApoB100 from Human HepG2 Cells." *J Nutr* 133(3): 700–706.

Palamara, A. T., L. Nencioni, K. Aquilano, et al. 2005. "Inhibition of Influenza A Virus Replication by Resveratrol." *J Infect Dis* 191(10): 1719–1729.

Palsamy, P., and S. Subramanian. 2008. "Resveratrol, a Natural Phytoalexin, Normalizes Hyperglycemia in Streptozotocin-Nicotinamide Induced Experimental Diabetic Rats." *Biomed Pharmacother* 62(9): 598–605.

Parente, Matilde. 2009. *Resveratrol*. Salt Lake City, UT: Woodland Publishing.

Queen, B. L., and T. O. Tollefsbol. 2010. "Polyphenols and Aging." *Curr Aging Sci* 3(1): 34–42.

Querfurth, Henry, and Frank LaFeria. 2010. "Alzheimer's Disease." *N Eng J Med* 362:329–344.

Sabbagh, Marwan Noel. 2008. *The Alzheimer's Answer: Reduce Your Risk and Keep Your Brain Healthy*. Hoboken, NJ: John Wiley and Sons.

Sakamoto, T., H. Horiguchi, E. Oguma, and F. Kayama. 2009. "Effects of Diverse Dietary Phytoestrogens on Cell Growth, Cell Cycle, and Apoptosis in Estrogen-Receptor-Positive Breast Cancer Cells." *J Nutr Biochem* 21(9): 856–864.

Scarlatti, Francesca, Giusy Sala, Giulia Somenzi, et al. 2003. "Resveratrol Induces Growth Inhibition and Apoptosis in Metastatic Breast Cancer Cells via De Novo Ceramide Signaling." *FASEB J* 17:2339–2341.

Schroecksnadel, K., C. Winkler, B. Wirleitner, et al. 2005. "Anti-inflammatory Compound Resveratrol Suppresses Homocysteine Formation in Stimulated Human Peripheral Blood Mononuclear Cells In Vitro." *Clin Chem Lab Med* 43(10): 1084–1088.

Solfrizzi, V., A. D'Introno, A. M. Colacicco, et al. 2007. "Alcohol Consumption, Mild Cognitive Impairment, and Progression to Dementia." *Neurology* 68:1790–1799.

Sönmez, U., A. Sönmez, G. Erbil, I. Tekmen, and B. Baykara. 2007. "Neuroprotective Effects of Resveratrol Against Traumatic Brain Injury in Immature Rats." *Neurosci Lett* 402(2): 133–137.

Stef, G., A. Csiszar, K. Lerea, Z. Ungvari, and G. Veress. 2006. "Resveratrol Inhibits Aggregation of Platelets from High-Risk Cardiac Patients with Aspirin Resistance." *J Cardiovasc Pharmacol* 48(2): 1–5.

Sun, C., Y. Hu, X. Liu, et al. 2006. "Resveratrol Downregulates the Constitutional Activation of Nuclear Factor-kappaB in Multiple Myeloma Cells, Leading to Suppression of Proliferation and Invasion, Arrest of Cell Cycle, and Induction of Apoptosis." *Cancer Genet Cytogenet* 165(1): 9–19.

Szkudelska, Katarzyna, and Tomasz Szkudelski. 2010. "Resveratrol, Obesity, and Diabetes." *Eur J Pharmacol* 635(1–3): 1–8.

Tessier, Peter. 2010. "Resveratrol Selectively Remodels Soluble Oligomers and Fibrils of Amyloid A into Off-pathway Conformers." *J Biol Chem* 285:24228–24237.

University of Alabama at Birmingham. 2007. "Red Wine Compound Shown to Prevent Prostate Cancer." News release, Aug. 31. http://main.it.uab.edu/Sites/MediaRelations/articles/38276.

University of Pittsburgh Cancer Institute. 2008. "Plant Antioxidant May Protect Against Radiation Exposure." News release, Sept. 23. www.upci.upmc.edu/news/upci_news/092308_plant.cfm.

University of Queensland. 2009. "Red Wine Ingredient Demonstrates Significant Health Benefits: Research Review." News release, June 12. www.uq.edu.au/news/?article=18573.

University of Rochester Medical Center. 2008. "Cigarettes Leave Deadly Path by Purging Protective Genes." News release, Jan. 17. www.urmc.rochester.edu/news/story/index.cfm?id=1838.

———. 2008. "Mounting Evidence Shows Red Wine Antioxidant Kills Cancer." News release, March 26. www.urmc.rochester.edu/news/story/index.cfm?id=1934.

University of Texas Southwestern Medical Center. 2009. "Study Shows How Substance in Grapes May Squeeze Out Diabetes." News release, Oct. 15. www.utsouthwestern.edu/utsw/cda/dept353744/files/555627.html.

University of Wisconsin School of Medicine and Public Health. 2009. "Uncorking a Wine-Related Cancer Treatment." News release, Jan. 22. www.med.wisc.edu/news-events/news/wine-related-cancer-treatment/308.

Vingtdeux, Valérie, Ute Dreses-Werringloer, Haitian Zhao, Peter Davies, and Philippe Marambaud. 2008. "Therapeutic Potential of Resveratrol in Alzheimer's Disease." *BMC Neuroscience* 9(Suppl 2): S6.

Wade, Nicholas. 2008. "Hoping Two Drugs Carry a Side Effect: Longer Life." *New York Times,* July 22.

———. 2010. "Potential Found in a New Approach to Alzheimer's." *New York Times,* July 23.

Wang, L. X., A. Heredia, H. Song, et al. 2004. "Resveratrol Glucuronides as the Metabolites of Resveratrol in Humans: Characterization, Synthesis, and Anti-HIV Activity." *J Pharm Sci* 93(10): 2448–2457.

Wood, L. G., P. A. Wark, and M. L. Garg. 2010. "Antioxidant and Anti-inflammatory Effects of Resveratrol in Airway Diseases." *Antiox Redox Signal*, March 9 (Epub ahead of print).

Wu, J. M. 2001. "Mechanism of Cardioprotection by Resveratrol, a Phenolic Antioxidant Present in Red Wine (Review)." *Int J Mol Med* 8(1): 3–17.

Xu, Y. 2010. "Antidepressant-like Effect of Trans-Resveratrol: Involvement of Serotonin and Noradrenaline System." *Eur Neuropsychopharmacol* 20(6): 405–413.

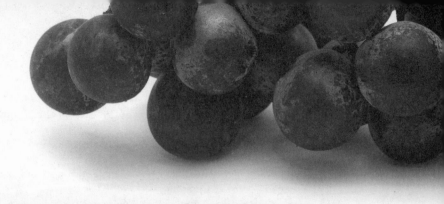

Acknowledgments

y thanks go to the many researchers who are advancing our ability to live longer, more healthful lives. In particular, I would like to acknowledge these resveratrol researchers: Dr. Lenny Guarente, Dr. David Sinclair, and Dr. Joseph Baur.

Special thanks go to Dr. Joseph Maroon for granting permission to use some information from his book, *The Longevity Factor*. Thanks also to journalist Nicholas Wade for his ongoing coverage of resveratrol.

Finally, I want to express my appreciation to the fantastic team of professionals at Book Publishing Company.

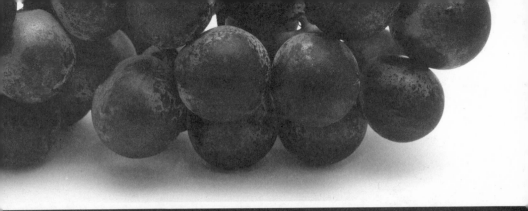

Index

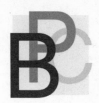

BOOK PUBLISHING COMPANY
since 1974—books that educate, inspire, and empower

To find sprouting seeds and other vegan favorites online, visit:
www.healthy-eating.com

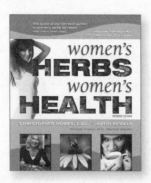

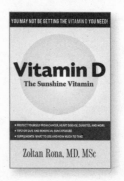

Women's Herbs, Women's Health
Christopher Hobbs, LAc,
Kathi Keville
978-1-57067-152-4 $24.95

Vitamin D
Zoltan Rona, MD, MSc
978-0-920470-82-4 $9.95

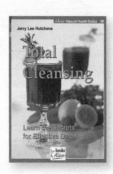

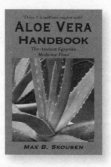

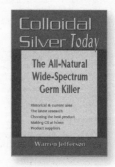

Total Cleansing
Jerry Lee Hutchens
978-1-55312-004-5
$11.95

Aloe Vera Handbook
Max B. Skousen
978-1-57067-169-2
$3.95

Colloidal Silver Today
Warren Jefferson
978-1-57067-154-8
$6.95

Purchase these health titles and cookbooks from your local bookstore or natural food store,
or you can buy them directly from:

Book Publishing Company • P.O. Box 99 • Summertown, TN 38483 • 1-800-695-2241

Please include $3.95 per book for shipping and handling.